CW00838979

The Fiber Factor

THE FIBER FACTOR

how to stay healthy with bran and high-fiber foods

from the staff of Prevention magazine
edited by Anne Moyer

Rodale Press, Inc., Emmaus, Pennsylvania 18049

Copyright © 1976 Rodale Press, Inc.

All rights reserved. No part of this publication may be reproduced or transmitted in any form or by any means, electronic or mechanical, including photocopy, recording, or any information storage and retrieval system without the written permission of the Publisher.

Printed in the United States of America on recycled paper

Library of Congress Cataloging in Publication Data
The Fiber factor: how to stay healthy with bran and high-fiber foods.

   Includes bibliographical references and index.
   1. Fiber deficiency diseases. 2. High-fiber diet.
3. Food—Fiber content. I. Moyer, Anne. II. Prevention.
RC627.F5F54   613.2'8   76-18923

ISBN 0-87857-127-2
2 4 6 8 10 9 7 5 3 1

Contents

Introduction

Humanity has come a long way since the first *Homo sapien* appeared on earth. We have organized ourselves into social groups, each of which has built up its own cultural patterns. Some groups, such as the Bantus in Africa and the Maoris in New Zealand, have chosen to live close to nature, without artifice. Other social groups, particularly in the West, have become "civilized," surrounding themselves with immensely complex industrial, economic, and political structures. In the West, we do not live as the land allows, but rather, we mold the world to our own wishes.

In industrial societies, people do not grow their own food, make their own clothes, or build their own dwellings. These basic tasks are all performed by industry, to allow us more time for leisure and recreation. We enjoy all the conveniences, all the amenities of civilized life, it's true, but now we are learning the price of our greed and laziness. We are paying for our easy lives with our health.

Intestinal disease of all kinds used to be rare. Now it runs rampant through the Western world, and it's increasing at a dizzying rate. We have run out of scapegoats to blame for our sickness, and we're start-

ing to find out that it's our own fault—a consequence
of tampering with our food. The refining processes we
believed so improved our flour and sugar have in
reality been destroying these basic foods and our
digestive systems along with them.

Refining removes from foods an absolutely vital
component we need to maintain intestinal health. This
substance is lost to us completely when we eat refined
flour and sugar products, because "enriching" and
"fortifying" don't put it back in. The vital factor
whose absence is ruining our digestive tracts is fiber—
you may know it as roughage, or bulk.

In recent years, medical researchers have discovered that the scarcity of fiber in the Western diet is
the key factor behind the soaring rates of bowel
disease in the Western world. They bring us the good
news that putting more fiber in our diets can put an
end to those skyrocketing statistics. And best of all,
the most effective, cheapest, easiest to use source of
the fiber we need so badly is a readily available, long-
forgotten substance we routinely refine out of our
flour—wheat bran. Bran is the outer portion of the
wheat kernel which is removed from the grain when it
is milled into white flour. Using whole grain flour
products (with bran intact) or simply adding bran to
the foods you now eat can protect you from colon
cancer, diverticulitis, chronic constipation, diabetes,
obesity, varicose veins, hemorrhoids, hiatus hernia,
peptic ulcer, diarrhea, gallstones, and even heart
disease. Believe it or not, all of these illnesses have
been shown to be direct or indirect results of the inef-
ficiency of our digestive and eliminatory systems
brought on by our refined-food diets.

The news about bran is revolutionary—to think a

single, simple dietary factor could be in such a large measure responsible for so many of our most widespread, most complex, and most serious health problems! The bran story fills us with hope—natural drugless remedies that really work are hard to find in our pharmaceutical society. And bran is an easily accessible remedy as well—simple to use, available in great quantity, and affordable by everybody. In our opinion, the bran treatment ranks among the most significant achievements in health care of the decade.

It is difficult, at first, to understand why it has taken so long for the good news about high-fiber foods to be heard. For one thing, there is great resistance from the food industry, at the moment, toward promoting the kinds of foods that will encourage bowel health. They are too cheap and don't require enough processing to provide a sufficient profit margin.

Further, the mass media might find themselves in trouble with all their food industry and laxative advertisers if they were to stress the value of eating whole, fresh foods and inexpensive bran.

But most startling of all is the reluctance of the medical profession to acknowledge the demonstrated benefits of increased fiber in the diet. The word about bran has been out for years—Dr. Thomas Cleave was reporting his successful use of bran over 30 years ago—but only in the past year has bran begun to receive the attention it deserves. Perhaps the medical profession is afraid to admit that its pet treatment for diverticulosis and other intestinal ailments, the low-residue diet, is counterproductive in many cases.

Fortunately for all of us, a small group of dedicated medical researchers refuse to disregard their findings merely because they contradict traditional medical practice. Their determined, outspoken support of high-fiber food has opened a new way for all of us to help ourselves to better health.

Not surprisingly, the spread of the bran story has spawned a flurry of new books on the subject. All these books were written to bring the news about bran to everyone—to those of us who don't get a chance to read the medical journals where this research first came to light. These books tell the bran story, but they don't always tell the whole story or keep it in perspective. Bran works in many ways; it does far more, for example, than stabilize body weight; but on the other hand, bran cannot work miracles. What bran offers is a steady, step-by-step improvement in health which eventually adds up to protection from many major diseases.

Now that the initial emotional reaction to the bran story has passed, it is time to consider objectively just what the new discoveries mean. Admittedly, bran does take getting used to. For a few weeks you may be somewhat uncomfortable with bran, until your digestive system becomes accustomed to functioning as it should. But we believe the rewards are more than worth the small discomfort. This book is intended to tell you what bran can and cannot do; how the addition to your diet of food fiber in all its forms (remember, bran is certainly not the only source of fiber) can help keep you from ever falling victim to the diseases of civilization or, if you already suffer intestinal problems, can help relieve your symptoms to make your disorder easier to live with. We believe you should know what actually happens inside your digestive tract and circulatory system when each of the diseases of civilization strikes and just how bran works in your intestines to solve the problem.

1 | Being Civilized Is A Pain in the ----!

Time was when the mention of the word "civilized" brought to mind an advanced culture in which science brought health and happiness to everyone and humanity was freed of many age-old afflictions.

Things have changed. Now that nearly everybody on earth has been exposed to the effects of civilization, people have begun to look around and wonder whether it was all worth it. Formerly pristine, unspoiled settings have yielded to civilized man's technology, only to end up on the brink of ruin, scarred with the filth of pollution and endangered by toxic industrial wastes.

But perhaps the most significant effect of civilization upon humanity, now established by doctors who specialize in epidemiology (the study of the distribution of diseases), is that many of our most familiar diseases come into being among primitive peoples only as they grow more civilized. The reason? As we have changed our pace of living, we have also changed our eating habits. We have begun to eat refined foods to the exclusion of whole, natural foods and the nutrients

1

they provide. In other words, the price of living and eating as a civilized person today is suffering and dying by a civilized person's diseases.

The so-called diseases of Western civilization encompass a wide range of noninfectious illnesses including digestive tract disorders such as diverticulosis, colon cancer, and gallbladder disease; cardiovascular problems such as ischemic heart disease (insufficient supply of blood to the heart caused by constriction of a blood vessel), hemorrhoids, varicose veins, phlebitis and deep vein thrombosis; and other metabolism-related ailments such as obesity and diabetes. These illnesses used to be regarded as unavoidable consequences of growing old, until the discovery that bran offers protection from their debilitating effects.

Bowel disease has spread rapidly in the last 50 years. So rampant is it that in medical circles, colon disease is regarded as a problem of great magnitude. A few years ago, Dr. William Seaman, Director of the Radiology Service at Columbia-Presbyterian Medical Center in New York, told radiologists that the common forms of colon disease "constitute a public health problem of immense proportion."[1]

There are two facts about this tremendous "public health problem" which all of us must face. One is that these ailments absolutely did not exist before the twentieth century except in very rare instances. For example, in 1900, diverticulosis was practically unknown; in 1920, it was not even in medical textbooks. But within 70 years, the current average life span of man, it has become the most common disorder of the colon in Western countries.

The second fact is that most forms of bowel disease, at least the nonmalignant types, can be controlled, and in most cases completely prevented, by a few simple dietary modifications. This means that lots of painful and costly surgery can be avoided and that now we can all be free of the intestinal discomforts so many of us have come to accept as "normal."

Dr. Denis P. Burkitt, an eminent British surgeon who spent 20 years in Uganda, observed some years ago the probable link between diet and intestinal disorders. He discovered that bowel disease is almost unknown among rural Africans. Yet in the United States and other Western nations, colon cancer accounts for 12 to 14 percent of all cancers. During his entire time in Africa, Dr. Burkitt did not encounter a single case of diverticulitis. The cause, he is convinced, is the difference in the kinds of foods eaten. This is no freak of geography either, because Africans who live in cities and eat Westernized diets soon begin to have as much bowel trouble as do the Englishmen who live in those same cities and who eat a strictly Western diet.

The rural African eats a diet which is high in indigestible food fiber, or roughage. His grain is refined only by minimal hand pounding with stones and so retains much of the outer covering, or bran, which is altogether removed from the white flour eaten by Westerners. He eats large amounts of fruit, vegetables, seeds, and roots, all of which are also rich in indigestible fiber. All of this fiber may offer him no nutrients, but when it reaches his lower intestine, it's a positive blessing—his digestive tract functions quickly and efficiently.

Now let's look at the average Westerner's diet. Traditionally, bread has been a major source of dietary fiber, but the white bread consumed in the "civi-

lized" portions of the world contains only a tiny fraction of the fiber present in the whole, unmilled wheat
berry. When the milling process removes the bran and
germ from the grain, 81.5 percent of the fiber goes
with them (according to *Composition of Foods*, USDA
Agriculture Handbook No. 8). In terms of bread, this
means you must eat eight or nine slices of white bread
to consume the amount of fiber you get in a single slice
of whole grain bread!

Of course, we all know that man can't live by
white bread alone, so what else does our average
Westerner eat? For one thing, he puts away astounding amounts of sugar. Over 100 pounds of it a year!
And he may not even realize when he's consuming
sugar, for it's an all-but-hidden ingredient in many
unsweet foods. Read a few labels in any supermarket
and you'll find sugar in a multitude of unlikely
products from meat tenderizers to canned peas.

According to USDA statistics, the average
American in 1970 consumed 264 pounds of empty-
calorie foods—102 pounds of table sugar, 88 pounds
of white flour, 53 pounds of refined fats and oils, 14
pounds of corn sugar, and 7 pounds of white rice.
These fattening foods made up over *half* of his total
food intake (calculated on the basis of dry weight),
and they contain only the slightest traces of fiber.

Americans today are also eating far more animal
fats (meat, fish, poultry, eggs, and dairy products)
than did our grandparents and great-grandparents.
These foods have no fiber *at all*.

At the same time, many foods that do have lots of
fiber—whole grain flour and cereal, whole potatoes,
fresh fruit and vegetables—are no longer an important part of our diets as they were in earlier times.

Our intake of whole wheat flour, bran, and similar products has dropped to a fifth or even a tenth of what it was in 1900. Consumption of dried beans, another good source of fiber, has also fallen sharply. Apples, potatoes, cabbage, and all the rest have as much fiber as they always had, but we are simply not eating as much of these foods as did our ancestors (see table 1).

TABLE 1
TRENDS IN ANNUAL PER CAPITA FOOD AVAILABILITY

	1909-13	1925-39	1947-49	1957-59	1965
Meat, poultry & fish, lbs	172	149	176	192	203
Eggs, lbs	37	36	47	45	39
Dairy products, qts	177	202	236	240	237
Fats and oils, lbs	59	66	57	57	57
Fruit, lbs	176	199	208	183	168
Potatoes, lbs	205	147	123	110	101
Other vegetables	203	232	232	209	208
Flour and cereals, lbs	291	204	171	148	147
Sugar and sweeteners, lbs	89	110	110	106	112

SOURCE: B. Friend, *American Journal of Clinical Nutrition* 20 (1967): 907.

This highly refined diet gives the digestive system less work to do, and the food passes through the intestinal tract quite slowly (it takes more than three days for the average Englishman to pass his food, compared to a mere 35 hours for a rural African). The exceedingly long time it takes food to travel through our intestines has been verified by a number of simple experiments which we'll discuss in "The Simple Answer to Constipation."

Another significant factor in determining the efficiency of intestinal function is the amount of solid waste excreted. There is a big difference in the weight of stools among Africans and Westerners. Dr. Burkitt found that Africans averaged 470 grams per stool. Two groups eating a diet of partly refined and partly unprocessed foods had an average of 200 grams per bowel movement. But the typical Englishman expelled only 108 grams per stool.

Many rural Africans, particularly those who eat primarily cornmeal and beans, produce such a great quantity of stool that they have two bowel movements each day and become quite concerned if they miss one.

Scientific research has produced impressive evidence that a decrease in intake of dietary fiber interferes with the operation of the intestines. Faulty intestinal function, in turn, is believed to influence the development of such conditions as obesity, diverticulitis, varicose veins, and the other diseases of Western civilization.

Available data show that where a low incidence of these diseases is present, a high intake of dietary fiber is also present. Adequate fiber insures consumption of fewer calories, faster passage of food through the gastrointestinal tract, greater weight of stool, bulkier stools which reduce strain and pressure in the colon, increased numbers of helpful fecal bacteria, and lower levels of cholesterol in the blood due to a change in the metabolism of bile salts.

Two other "civilized" diseases—diabetes and obesity—are now believed to be largely caused by consumption of refined, concentrated starches and sugars. Dr. Burkitt and other prominent medical experts insist that consuming too much sugar and too little fiber are both devastating results of the practice of refining carbohydrate foods. Our bodies were designed for and have long been accustomed to getting carbohydrates (the nutrient we need for energy) in small doses, accompanied by liberal amounts of fiber. But since the advent of refining, we have exposed our bodies to large quantities of naked, concentrated energy food that is rapidly absorbed into our blood. The onslaught of all these carbohydrates exerts a severe strain on the insulin-producing cells in the pancreas. If the body's insulin supplies become too unbalanced, diabetes will result. (See "How to Overcome Obesity and Defeat Diabetes" for the full story.)

The major sources of carbohydrates in the average Western diet are sucrose (refined sugar) and white flour—both of which are stripped of fiber during refining. Because most of us have grown up with these foods as part of our customary diet, it's difficult for us to realize how unnatural such foods are and that our bodies are just not equipped to handle them in large amounts.

We generally regard carbohydrates as fattening—in fact, most reducing diets restrict them. But primitive societies consume more than twice as much carbohydrates as we do, yet there are practically no obese members of these societies, and almost half the adults in the United States and England are overweight. The African Bantu, for example, eats 580 grams of carbohydrates a day, but the Englishman averages only 220 grams per day. So why do the British grow fat while the Bantus remain lean? Of course, the Bantus get more exercise, but just as important, they eat their carbohydrate foods unrefined, with fiber intact. (To learn how it works, see "How to Overcome Obesity and Defeat Diabetes.")

Doctors seeking reasons for the climbing rates of

bowel disease in civilized countries are placing more and more of the blame on the drastic changes in Western diet in the last century. Although we may not realize it, our eating habits have, indeed, changed radically.

The introduction of the roller mill in England during the 1880s made possible on a large scale the removal of cereal fiber (bran) from wheat during the manufacture of white flour. The consumption of refined sugar in that country doubled around the same time. From then on, our intake of refined, low-roughage foods has steadily increased.

We in America have all too willingly accepted modern food technology without pausing to examine the possible dangers of a diet largely dependent on refined, heavily processed foods. Doctors are not adequately trained in nutrition, and many dieticians and nutritionists haven't considered the fact that processing destroys fiber or investigated the effects of a fiberless diet on man's intestinal tract. Until quite recently, very little had been written in contemporary medical and nutritional literature about our need for roughage.

The case for fiber has been stated quite convincingly by Dr. Burkitt: The diseases of Western civilization—colon cancer, diverticulitis, heart disease, gallstones, varicose veins, obesity—all have the same geographical distribution. In areas where these diseases occur frequently, people consume larger amounts of fat, protein, sugar, and other refined carbohydrates, and far less fiber in their daily diets than people in areas with a low incidence of these illnesses.

In the view of Dr. Burkitt and a steadily mounting number of his colleagues, the intermediary factor between a refined diet and many of the diseases of civilization is constipation. Constipation is now believed to combine with other factors to lead, in turn, to the more serious disorders encountered in Western societies. Here's why.

Despite physicians' assurances to the contrary, constipation is not a natural state for the bowels to function in. Decaying food wastes lying in the large intestine for abnormal lengths of time, followed by straining of the intestinal muscles to expel the small, hard stools, certainly does not encourage bowel health. We simply cannot expose our intestinal tracts to such abnormal conditions year after year without expecting our bodies to react in some way.

The currently popular practice of taking laxatives to eliminate the constipation does not help solve the problem; in fact, prolonged laxative use actually *causes* chronic constipation! The only way to truly cure constipation is to treat the cause, not just the symptoms. Now that our refined diet has been shown to be the chief cause of constipation, and constipation the cause of other diseases, we must look to high-fiber foods for relief of this basic ailment before we can hope to relieve the more serious ones.

At this point, you may well be wondering just what is so special about bran. The fact is, we all need to put some bran in our diets every single day, and the next chapter will explain why. As we explained before, bran and other fibrous foods won't work instant miracles. You cannot expect your intestinal tract to whip back into shape overnight. Like a rusty piece of machinery, your bowels (if you're eating the foods most Americans eat) are slow and creaky, and they haven't been operating properly for years. When you

oil the machinery, you allow time for the oil to lubri-
cate the parts before you expect the machinery to run
smoothly; in the same way, you must give bran a
chance to do its work before your bowels begin to
function efficiently as nature intended. Remember, it
took years of abuse for your bowels to become sluggish, so you must allow a fraction of that time to repair
the damage.

Bran stands out as the most effective and by far
the cheapest source of fiber around. And using bran is
convenient—you don't have to change your whole diet
to take advantage of its benefits. In the next chapter,
you'll learn more reasons why bran is the best source
of fiber you can use and what it does for you that no
other food can do as well.

2 | What Makes Bran So Special?

When millers began to remove the bran from wheat flour in the 1880s, no one had any reason to question the procedure. After all, bran has almost no nutritional value to humans, so why keep it in the flour? Now we're beginning to see why bran should have been kept in flour—we desperately need its fiber.

Before we get into the special properties of bran, perhaps we should backtrack a bit and define exactly what is meant by "dietary fiber."

First we should be aware that the physical appearance of a food offers no clues to the amount of fiber it contains. A chewy steak or roast may appear to be full of fiber, while a spoonful of whole wheat flour seems too smooth to have any fiber whatsoever. The term "fiber" denotes a group of complex carbohydrates, including cellulose, hemicellulose, lignin, and pectin, which pass through the entire gastrointestinal tract without being broken down by enzymes. These substances are found only in plant foods.

Meat and dairy products do not contain any fiber at all. The toughest piece of meat or gristle, even if you cannot chew it, will be acted upon by the enzymes and gastric juices of your digestive system. Bones, too, if ground or crushed between the teeth, can be digested in the human body.

On the other hand, the fibers in whole plant foods cannot be altered by any digestive enzyme and pass intact through the gastrointestinal tract to form bulk in the lower intestine. Fibrous materials make up the cell walls and other structural formations within plants.

In whole, unprocessed carbohydrate foods, each starch-containing cell is surrounded by an envelope of fiber. This is the form in which our bodies were meant to accept carbohydrates. The modern refining process, however, breaks down the cell walls to expose the starchy interior, then removes the fiber, leaving "naked" carbohydrates. Our gastrointestinal tract was not designed to handle carbohydrates without their protective fiber coverings—in nature, starch is not found naked. And our modern bowel problems bear witness to the unnaturalness of our refined foods.

Fruit, vegetables, and grains all contain fiber. As a rule, unrefined foods contain far more fiber than refined foods. The refining process, as we said, strips foods of this valuable component. For example, whole wheat bread contains the fiber present in all parts of the wheat berry, but white bread has had the fibrous portions of the wheat kernel removed (see Appendix B). Fruit like apples also offer roughage, particularly in the skins, but when these fruit are canned or baked into pies, most of the fiber is destroyed. Generally speaking, grain foods are better suppliers of roughage to the diet. The fiber in fruit and vegetables is softer and begins to break down when these foods are cooked; part of it is digested in your stomach.

Unprocessed wheat bran stands out above other grain products as our best source of dietary fiber for several reasons. Bran is 85 percent dry material, but it has the property of absorbing large amounts of water—it will soak up eight to nine times its own volume. It is this water that makes the large, soft stool that passes easily. Other fibrous foods, such as nuts, cannot match the absorptive ability of bran.

Also, bran is a highly concentrated form of fiber. It is approximately 12 percent crude fiber, which is about five times the amount in whole wheat. You can include bran in your meals every day without causing a major change in your dietary pattern. Luckily, bran is almost tasteless, having a somewhat dry flavor, much like you might imagine a little sawdust would taste. It can be added to soups, sauces, and many other dishes without affecting the flavor of the food. If you bake, you can easily add it to muffins or bread. If you eat cereal for breakfast, add some bran to it. Or sprinkle bran on your buttered toast. (For recipes and other suggestions, see "Eating Bran Can Be Grand.")

Another advantage of bran over such sources of fiber as nuts, dried fruit, and bread is that the calories (and other nutrients) in bran are absorbed only to a negligible extent. In fact, bran can even be a valuable reducing aid because while it contributes few, if any, calories, it helps give your stomach that filled feeling. Just 20 grams of bran has the bulking effect in your stomach of 200 to 300 grams of most whole foods, so it satisfies you much quicker.

Finally, because so much bran is made available by the refining of white flour, it is very inexpensive. However, the price goes up considerably when it is packaged and sold as a ready-to-eat cereal. Most such bran-based breakfast cereals also have two other

things wrong with them: they are not 100 percent unprocessed bran, which is the kind of bran used in the
successful medical studies, and most of them come
mixed with sugar (see Appendix C). Sugar is just what
you want to avoid.

As bran doesn't have much market appeal or
profit potential, supermarkets seldom, if ever, carry
it. Most health food stores do carry bran, but if your
local store does not stock it, you can tell the proprietor
that it is available from at least two national distribu-
tors—Shiloh Farms (Route #59, Sulphur Springs,
Arizona, 72768) and Village Market (Box 546,
Boyertown, Pennsylvania, 19512). Or you can order
bran directly from Walnut Acres, Penns Creek,
Pennsylvania, 17862.

No one has yet established a specific amount of
dietary fiber which is ideal, and no one ever will. Dr.
Neil S. Painter and his colleagues (see chapter 8) discovered that the amount of bran which their patients
required to abolish their irritable bowel symptoms
varied greatly. The amount their patients took ranged
from one dessertspoon (about 3 grams) daily to three
tablespoons three times daily. The average was about
two teaspoons three times a day (a total of about 12
grams), but you must find your own optimal amount.
How much bran is best for you will depend on your intake of fiber from other sources, such as fresh vegetables and whole grain breads. The best way to determine how much bran you need is to begin with one
or two teaspoons a day and gradually increase the
amount of bran until the desired effect takes hold.

When you begin to add bran to your diet, you will
probably find that it causes some flatulence and
distension. But don't allow this temporary discomfort

to stop you from taking bran, because in most cases it will disappear within two or three weeks. It takes about that long for your bowels to become accustomed to functioning as they should. So start out slowly and give your system a chance to get used to bran.

Some people object to bran on the ground that it is scratchy. But when bran is moistened, it is no longer scratchy at all. In your intestines, bran soaks up liquid like a sponge, and the roughage turns into "softage." Be sure to take your bran with fluids. Bran can't do its job without enough water to moisten it.

A few people, such as those with intestinal stenosis or adhesions, will not be able to tolerate bran at all. These people will probably find that fiber from fruit, vegetables, and whole grains, though not as convenient, will do the trick.

Fresh fruit such as apples, peaches, plums, and pears, if eaten with skins intact, are all good sources of fiber and contain a lot of water as well. Fruit with seeds, such as strawberries and raspberries, as well as prunes and figs, are also high in fiber. Bananas, cantaloupe, persimmons, and tomatoes offer fiber as well. Of course, you should avoid fruit that has been sprayed with insecticides. If unsprayed fruit is not available, soak the fruit for a few minutes in one-quarter cup of vinegar diluted in a dishpan of water, and then rinse the fruit in clear water. This will remove 85 percent of the surface spray.

Fresh leafy green vegetables, such as cabbage, lettuce, beet greens, and spinach, are valuable fiber foods as are foods rich in unrefined starch, such as white potatoes, sweet potatoes, pumpkins, squash, and carrots. Other vegetables that promote healthy bowel action are string beans, bean sprouts, brussels sprouts, broccoli, asparagus, celery, and avocados. Remember to cook vegetables only until they are fork tender—never let them get mushy. Cooking vegetables only a short time preserves more of their nutritional content and leaves more of their fiber intact. Better yet, eat them raw whenever possible.

Dried fruits are also an excellent source of fiber, but they should be taken with plentiful fluids, soaked or stewed. For additional fiber, boil potatoes in their skins and eat a fresh salad each day.

As we noted earlier, whole grains provide even better sources of fiber than fruit and vegetables. So, instead of buying breakfast cereal that is sugar coated, fruit flavored, puffed, popped or otherwise tampered with, opt for unsugared granola, good old-fashioned oatmeal, and similarly unprocessed cereals. Empty your cupboards of fluffy, flavorless white bread and stock them instead with chewy, delicious breads and muffins made from whole grain wheat, rye, corn, and oats that have been stone-ground. You might even enjoy baking your own bread, and whole grain flours are available in most health food stores and even in some supermarkets. If you do buy commercially packaged breads, check the labels to make sure their darker color comes from the presence of whole grains and not artificial colors. Perhaps you would also like to experiment with making your own corn pones and hush puppies from whole cornmeal. And treat yourself to brown rice instead of polished white rice—it has a rich nutty flavor.

All these fiber-rich foods will be a big plus in your diet. Whether or not you can include bran too, these foods will get you away from the empty-calorie-naked-carbohydrate syndrome and take you back to the pure and simple foods your body was meant to thrive on.

Now that you know why you need bran, it's time to examine the problem of the diseases of civilization and take a look at how bran can help relieve them. The logical place to begin is with constipation—the first indication most people have that all is not well with their bowels.

Constipation is not the trifle it was once thought to be, especially if it continues for any length of time. Prolonged constipation is often the first warning signal that more serious problems are developing in the intestinal tract. Or the constipation itself can be the cause of ailments that may seem to have nothing to do with the intestinal tract (varicose veins, for example).

In order to protect yourself from the dangerous diseases of civilization, you must first understand and avoid constipation. The following chapter will show you the way.

3 The Simple Answer To Constipation

The digestive tract of modern man is something like the New York subway system at 5:30 P.M. when the tracks have just been hit by a power failure. Some trains are derailed, the tubes fill with noxious fumes from smoldering electrical fires, and passenger cars pile up by the dozens and hundreds behind paralyzed switches.

Translate passenger cars as food waste and you have a very good picture of what happens in the large intestines of many Americans on an almost daily basis. And just as many New Yorkers have become brutally conditioned to the point where they accept such transit nightmares as normal, so many Americans have come to accept irregularity, blockages, cramps, and near-unbearable discomfort as part of the "normal" operation of their intestinal transit systems. After all, if it wasn't "normal," why would there be so many ads for laxatives on the mass media? Why would the shelves of drugstores be chockablock with laxatives of every size, potency, color, and flavor?

Constipation afflicts Americans of all ages, sizes,

and income groups; we spend $200 million a year on the laxatives we depend on to relieve it, and yet, many doctors consider constipation so unimportant that they neglect its treatment and fail to seek out its causes. The unfortunate patient who complains of not having had a bowel movement in two or three days is reassured that this is a normal state of affairs for a middle-aged person. And if things get too bad, just use a laxative or enema. This answer to constipation is comforting and simple, but it is the wrong answer. Constipation must *not* be dismissed as a normal state of affairs, and a closer look at how it happens will explain why.

In order to comprehend what goes wrong in constipated bowels, it is first necessary to understand how the healthy intestinal system functions. Although it's been shown that less will do, nature has provided us with 20 to 25 feet of small intestine. Unimpressively shaped like a sausage, it does the impressive job of breaking down and converting foods so they can be utilized by tissues and organs. Using from one to two pints of bile from the liver, aided by an equal amount of digestive fluid from the pancreas and five to ten quarts of secretion daily from its own 20 million minute glands, the small intestine converts starch into glycogen, proteins into amino acids, and fat into fatty acids.

Moved by peristaltic muscles, food passes through the intestine tube at a slow rate, stopping every few inches for periods of up to 30 minutes, allowing a complex of muscles to disintegrate the food by churning. As this process continues, the intestine's lining absorbs digested proteins and carbohydrates into the bloodstream and fats into the lymphatic system, leaving the remainder of mucus and dead cells, a gruel, to be passed on to the large intestine.

Progress is slower in the large intestine, the gruel requiring three to four hours to travel through its five- or six-foot length. Unlike the small intestine, the large one abounds with friendly bacteria that manufacture B and K vitamins. The large intestine or colon, as it is known, extracts water and salts from the gruel, which are needed to properly maintain the body's mineral and fluid balance.

Depleted of nutrients and much of its fluid, the residue passes on to the rectum—the lower six inches of the colon—where its presence triggers the defecation reflex, and we become conscious of our need to expel the waste.

Constipation means, of course, that bowel movements are dry and hard to pass or bowel action occurs so infrequently that uncomfortable symptoms develop. But how does it actually occur? We have a natural reflex to promote expulsion of the rectal contents. Known as the *gastrocolic reflex*, it is triggered when the stomach or first part of the small intestine becomes distended by food or liquid. This is why people normally feel the urge to pass stool after eating. In constipation, the gastrocolic reflex isn't triggered as often as it should be, and food wastes remain in the rectum.

The idea of what constitutes regularity has touched off a great deal of controversy. Traditionally, symptoms of constipation—nausea, headache, abdominal discomfort—were believed due to "autointoxication," or absorption of poisons from the fecal matter. Although that belief was long ago disproved, contemporary medical research makes a strong case for the necessity of prompt evacuation of food wastes on the grounds that the human intestine was never meant to be a holding tank for food waste and allowing it to become one is inviting disease and infection. Chronic constipation has been shown to be a forerunner to severe intestinal ailments such as diverticulitis, venous disorders including hemorrhoids and varicose veins, heart attacks, and even cancer of the colon.

On the other hand, many doctors feel that in some people, particularly those who may be very sedentary, of an older age, or who simply don't eat very much, there is nothing at all abnormal about having only two or three bowel movements a week— perhaps even fewer in some cases. Unless the patient is suffering from a feeling of distress as a result of these infrequent movements or has painful bowel movements in which hard, dry stools are passed, he or she may not be constipated at all. According to this second school of thought, the patient is simply on his or her own schedule. Still, we take in food each day, we digest food each day, so is it not only logical that we should also expel wastes each day?

In general, we can say that there are three basic kinds of constipation. One is what doctors call "organic" in nature; that is, caused by a specific bodily condition such as a physical blockage, injury, or disease. Organic constipation can be caused by serious ailments such as cancer of the colon, ureteral stones, amebic colitis, liver and gallbladder diseases, anal fissures, or disorders of the blood vessels in the abdominal area. Ulcers or thrombosed hemorrhoids prevent relaxation of the anal sphincter, but such injuries are more likely to be a *result* of constipation— through straining—rather than a cause.

Drugs can also bring on organic constipation. All medications, such as opiates, designed to slow down nerve reactions can be constipating. For example, paregoric, which is given for diarrhea, is camphorated tincture of opium. Certain nonabsorbable antacid preparations can also create constipation.

Although serious conditions must not always be ruled out as causes of constipation, sometimes the medical problem may be as simple as weak stomach or back muscles, which may be caused by multiple pregnancies.

A second kind of constipation is due to stress encountered when living habits are changed radically. Usually, this type of constipation will appear during a vacation or business trip, when your daily routine is disrupted and you are in unfamiliar surroundings, or during brief periods of hospitalization.

The third general type of constipation is by far the most serious. Known as functional, or habitual, constipation, this variety generates most of the annual 200 million dollars' worth of laxative sales.

After transitory changes of habit and physical illness have been ruled out as causes of constipation, what is left? The two most common causes—which are often related—are psychologically induced failure of the normal defecation reflex and a diet lacking sufficient roughage.

Many psychological factors can interfere with the expression of the simple urge to move one's bowels. Some of the causes may stem back to childhood toilet training. Other people disrupt their normal defecation reflex by repeatedly failing to heed its call. After months or years of such a pattern of denial, the normal relationship between waste matter ready to move, nervous impulses, and muscular reactions leading to defecation is short-circuited. In many people, tension and worry can paralyze intestinal traffic by tensing those controlling nerves.

Lack of adequate fiber in the diet often occurs simultaneously with an impaired defecation reflex to cause constipation. Basically, fiber is needed to give bulk to the waste so that it can be promptly and easily moved by segmental wave activity through the colon (up, over, down and out). Mass propulsive movements normally occur once a day. But because the colon is much larger than the simple vessels designed to carry blood or urine and contains segments (something like a long string of sausages), waste matter must obviously have sufficient bulk to be moved through this system.

Actually, most of the bulk in a stool consists of water, not food or food residue. But the water must be absorbed by the residue, and here is the problem: fiberless food can't absorb enough water to move easily through the colon. No matter what volume of fiber-depleted food we eat, there is not enough residue for the water to be absorbed into in order to create the soft but firm bulk needed for easy elimination.

But what happens to the water in the bowels that is not absorbed by the food waste? It is simply reabsorbed by the body through the wall of the colon. This removal of water is quite a vigorous process, with the result that when scanty waste matter moves sluggishly through the bowels, even the small amount of water that it has managed to absorb can be removed from it and returned to the body. By the time waste matter reaches the rectum, it may be extremely compact and dry. It will also tend to be highly segmented and shaped by the contractions of the intestines. In contrast, waste matter which contains generous amounts of fiber, and therefore of water, tends to be large, soft, and unsegmented.

Clearly, the answer to this problem is to somehow introduce more bulk into the diet, particularly the kind of bulk that will absorb and hold great amounts of water.

HOW DOCTORS TREAT CONSTIPATION

Most patients who go into a doctor's office to seek help with constipation do so only after repeated but unsuccessful attempts to treat it themselves. But they are not automatically going to get the help they seek from their doctors. In fact, many doctors cannot be counted upon to give even strictly medical help. Dr. Norman D. Nigro of Wayne State University School of Medicine in Detroit told his fellow physicians at a panel presentation on constipation held at the 1974 American Medical Association (AMA) convention in Chicago that too many physicians lack adequate knowledge about either the significance or the proper management of constipation.

Doctors (and patients, too!) should be especially alert if the constipation appears relatively suddenly. After questioning the patient about possible changes in his life-style and giving him a physical examination, the doctor may perform a digital examination of the rectum. Finding only a few grams of feces in the rectum indicates that habitual constipation is present. The next logical step is to search for local lesions in the area of the anus and rectum. This is generally done with specialized tools such as the anoscope and sigmoidoscope. In many cases, X-rays and a barium enema will be administered, but to avoid putting barium above an obstructive lesion, the doctor must first visually examine the rectal area.

Constipation induced by habitual use of drugs, such as narcotics, antacid aluminum salts, phenothiazines, tricyclic antidepressants, and certain antihypertensive drugs, is usually treated with laxatives.

If constipation is due to a lack of urge to defecate, doctors often prescribe glycerin suppositories to stimulate bowel movement. If hard, dry stools are the problem, an oil retention enema at night, followed in the morning by either a glycerin suppository or a tap water enema, can encourage smoother and easier elimination. Stool softeners and bulk-producing agents can also help in cases of small, hard stools.

If these standard medical treatments fail to relieve the constipation, doctors may suggest surgery. Surgical treatments for constipation can range from anal repairs that require only local anesthesia to a complex resectioning of the colon necessitated by thickened intestinal muscles or volvulus (an obstruction of the intestine caused by the intestine twisting upon itself).

LAXATIVES DON'T SOLVE THE PROBLEM

More Americans are now suffering from constipation than ever before, and we're guzzling gallons of laxatives in an attempt to speed up our sluggish bowels. Americans are notorious for taking the easy way out. We want a pill for everything: to sleep soundly, to wake up brightly, to be happy, and even to have regular bowel movements. It's gotten to the point where we worry more about which laxative is best than about whether or not we need them at all! Even doctors are brainwashed on the subject.

The *Handbook of NonPrescription Drugs* (1973) of the American Pharmaceutical Association reports that more than 700 different laxative preparations are sold over the counter; in 1971, one percent of all physicians' prescriptions in the United States were for laxatives alone!

We need to take time out to consider just what all those laxatives are doing to us. Laxatives are habit forming, they're an unnecessary expense, and they may cause real harm to the body. Most importantly, there are far better and safer ways to prevent and cure constipation—we simply don't need laxatives!

People who rely on laxatives are exposing themselves to needless hazards. For in all but a very few cases, constipation is not truly present before the hang-up over "regularity" begins. When laxatives are taken every day or two to encourage regularity, they ao the exact opposite of what they're supposed to do—your intestinal muscles become so worn out from the constant stimulation that they grow flaccid and finally quit in exhaustion. Your natural gastrocolic reflex is no longer functioning, and now you actually cannot move your bowels without the laxative. Thus, the medication has in reality *caused* constipation, and you can't move your bowels normally.

In other words, it's the cart first and the horse in the rear. The patient assumes he's constipated when his bowels don't kick off like an alarm clock every morning. He panics, reaches for a laxative, and then he really becomes constipated

In addition to destroying your gastrocolic reflex, a strong laxative that "cleans out the system" removes not only waste matter that should normally have been eliminated that day but much of the still-liquid waste matter above it in the tract. Consequently, after such a purging, you find that you have no bowel movement for the next few days (it has been found that normal colonic activity stops for 48 hours after a strong laxative or purgative is taken) and take more laxatives because you believe you're still constipated.

Such complete emptying of the contents of the intestines also means that food is pushed through before it can be broken down and absorbed into the body. Thus, valuable nutrients are lost, and the patient taking laxatives on a regular basis can suffer from malnutrition. Also, the constant activity while the drug is working irritates intestinal membranes.

The constipation conscious have an array of chemical wares to choose from. Drugstore and supermarket shelves are crammed with laxatives that act in any one or more of the following ways: irritating the intestine to stimulate peristalsis (the muscular contractions which move wastes along), lubricating the intestine so wastes slide through more easily, softening the stool by boosting the amount of water in the intestine, and increasing bulk to form larger stools.[1]

Stimulants are probably the most dangerous of the laxative families. This kind of laxative irritates the intestine and, when taken in doses large enough to relieve constipation, can cause diarrhea, cramps, and fluid depletion. Habitual use of stimulants can result in chronic constipation, a dangerous depletion of the vital mineral potassium, malabsorption of nutrients in the intestine, and other disorders.

Among the more well-known stimulants are cascara, casanthranol, calomel, senna derivatives, danthron, aloe, phenolphthalein, and bisacodyl. These substances are contained singly and in various combinations in many over-the-counter and prescription laxative preparations, including Ex-Lax, Carter's Little Pills, Nature's Remedy, Dulcolax, Doxidan, and Senokot.

Castor oil also belongs to this group, being among the most irritating and fast acting of the stimulants. Prune juice can also be classified as a stimulant laxative, although the mechanism by which it works is not fully understood.

Despite all the well-documented ill effects of stimulant laxatives, they are still hard-sold to both the general public and doctors. One well-known senna product has for years been heavily advertised in major medical journals, and probably many patients are taking this harmful laxative on the recommendations of their own physicians!

Softener laxatives, also called lubricants, coat waste matter with a slick layer that permits it to slide quickly through the intestines. These products pass unaltered through the digestive tract and can hinder absorption of nutrients.

Probably the most common of the lubricants is mineral oil, which is also the most dangerous. Taking mineral oil orally can interfere with the absorption of food if taken with meals. It robs the body of the fat-soluble vitamins A, D, E, and K and impedes absorption of calcium and phosphorus. The *Medical Letter*, in a review of laxatives (November 23, 1973), warned that elderly and debilitated people are liable to develop a type of chemical pneumonia if they accidentally inhale mineral oil when vomiting or swallowing. Some doctors recommend taking it before going to bed or on an empty stomach, but why take chances? Avoid it completely.

A third type of laxative is the saline cathartic, or dehydrator. These mineral salt compounds draw water through the intestinal wall, dilute the fecal matter to an almost liquid state, and expel it. Dehydrators are made from such mineral compounds as magnesium sulfate and sodium biophosphate and include milk of magnesia USP, Epsom salts, Fleet's Phospho-Soda, and Sal Hepatica.

Laxatives containing magnesium are hazardous for many patients because magnesium ions are absorbed into other parts of the body from the intestine. In patients with impaired kidney function, the ions can accumulate and cause depression of the central nervous system. One popular magnesium product has been known to produce nosebleeds. So much sodium is often absorbed into the body from sodium-containing laxatives that patients with cardiovascular or similar disorders can develop edema, an accumulation of fluid in the tissues.

The main objection to the dehydrators is that the diarrhea they cause robs the body of important vitamins and minerals. Potassium is one of the minerals depleted by diarrhea, and the lack of it, when severe enough, leads to muscular weakness and even paralysis, a weakening of the heart muscle, severe intestinal gas, and decreased alkalinity of the blood and tissues associated with kidney failure.

A fourth category of laxatives, the bulk producers, includes agar, psyllium, and cellulose derivatives. These are the slowest acting laxatives; they swell in the intestine, much as a wet sponge would, and create added bulk that activates peristalsis, the mechanism for elimination.

Bulk producers have created some rather alarming situations when there was enough liquid in the intestines to make the preparation gummy but not enough water to soften it and allow it to mix with other bowel contents. When insufficient liquid is present, the bulk formers can cause fecal impaction, obstruction, and sometimes, intestinal perforation. There are two widely known bulk formers—Serutan and Metamucil.

Medical reports continue to add new dangers to the alarming list of already known side effects caused by laxatives. Two independent studies were simultaneously published in the *Journal of the American Medical Association* (January 5, 1970) reporting the outbreak of jaundice in two groups of patients using the patent formula Dialose Plus. Both research teams singled out the ingredient oxyphenisatin acetate as the culprit guilty of inflaming the liver.

Commenting editorially on both sides, the AMA said, "Oxyphenisatin acetate is a component of many laxative mixtures, some of them virtual polypharmacons (several drugs together) sold without prescription to laymen. Enough harm is done by over-the-counter laxatives without adding liver damage to the spectrum of damage." The editorial concluded: "The widespread marketing of a drug as trivial as a laxative, particularly over the counter, seems beyond justification if it has the potentiality for harm that has been shown with oxyphenisatin acetate."

In light of the fact that such huge quantities of laxatives are sold, it is clear that a self-perpetuating cycle is involved. Laxatives treat the symptoms but not the cause of constipation, and unless a change is made in diet and living habits, patients will continue to form the same small, hard, dry stools for which they originally took the drugs. As the symptoms continue, laxative use will also continue until, in time, patients feel they cannot have a bowel movement without taking a laxative. The stimulant-type laxatives are particularly addictive. A person becomes constipated, begins taking a stimulant laxative, and then becomes permanently constipated through the actual destruction of his normal defecation reflex, thereby becoming dependent on the laxative.

A dimension of psychological dependence also accompanies habitual laxative use. So strong is the mere *belief* that a laxative is necessary that the study cited in the *Medical Letter* found that 14 out of 20 patients with chronic constipation were able to have satisfactory bowel movements over a two-week period when treated with placebos instead of real laxatives.[2]

The first step in conquering constipation, then, is to throw out all the laxatives in the house and buy no more. You can't hope to have a normal bowel movement until you're free of their crippling effects.

Of course, for the chronic laxative user the period of transition following the discontinuation of the drug can be a difficult time. It takes courage to stop taking laxatives, just as it's hard to quit smoking or break any other bad habit. If you require help during the first few weeks, you might try giving yourself an enema. Use a pint of warm water containing a level teaspoon of table salt. Hold the enema bag about two feet above the toilet seat and let the water flow in gently. This should allow you to have a bowel movement, and it's somewhat better than using a laxative. But bear in mind that an enema will clean the upper as well as the lower bowel, stopping colon activity for hours. Don't make enemas a regular practice.

If you pay attention to developing normal bowel habits and avoid laxatives, you need never be constipated again. Laxatives are a crutch you can do without, and you'll be surprised that your gas pains, your irritability, and your indigestion will disappear after you stop taking them.

HOW TO GET RID OF YOUR CONSTIPATION

If laxatives aren't the way to cure constipation, what is the answer? There are many drugless treatments for constipation that get right at the cause of the problem instead of just relieving the symptoms.

First of all, it's a good idea to establish a regular time of day for evacuation, so that your body gets into the habit. Surprisingly, many people don't recognize the importance of developing their own regular elimination habits. And even though current medical opinion finds nothing wrong with irregular bowel habits, having a daily movement is still best if you want to avoid constipation and its complications.

Perhaps the most important advice is simply to heed the call when it comes. Like so many things in the body, the gastrocolic reflex works better the more you use it. On the other hand, if you fail to obey the normal urges it sends out, the signals will become weaker and weaker, and it will take larger and larger volumes of stool to trigger the urge. You may lose the reflex entirely and become severely constipated if you continue to ignore your body's call.

When you're in the bathroom try to relax and allow yourself plenty of time—at least 10 or 15 minutes—for the reflex to take effect. Remember, too, that squatting is the normal position for a bowel movement, but modern toilets don't take this into account. New design concepts show toilets much lower than the conventional flush model, but it will be quite a while before they gain public acceptance. Some people prefer to squat over a chamber pot rather than use a commode. At any rate, you'll find it easier to pass stool if you elevate your feet on a footstool in front of the toilet or else bend forward so that your abdomen rests against your thighs.

Teaching your bowels to move regularly is a little like teaching yourself to wake up at a given hour every morning. It can be done, and once you have learned to do it, the habit will persist.

HOW TO EAT FOR REGULARITY

Diet is probably the single most important factor in cases of constipation. Bowels are made sluggish chiefly by what you put into them. Some foods pass through the intestinal tract quickly and others get bogged down—it's as simple as that.

The residue of the food you eat is easier to eliminate if it contains roughage (fiber) to stimulate the colonic muscles and help form large, soft, easy-to-pass stools.

The refined foods so abundant in American supermarkets and kitchens are almost completely digested and absorbed, giving us too many calories and too little residue to pass easily. If you want to restore your regularity, you've first got to cut out heavily processed foods such as white breads (biscuits, rolls, hotcakes, pastries, cakes, doughnuts, etc.), refined pastas (spaghetti, macaroni, and noodles), sugary sweets, soft drinks, overcooked vegetables, gravies, rich sauces, and other lifeless foods.

Many experts maintain that the removal of nearly all the bran from flour in modern refining is only *part* of the reason why constipation is now one of the most common chronic diseases. The other reason is the huge increase which has occurred during the last hundred years in the consumption of *refined sugar*.

This increase in sugar consumption resulted in people fulfilling (often *over*fulfilling) their caloric requirements without eating the large amounts of bread, porridge, potatoes, cabbage, beans, and other fiber-rich foods which they previously relied upon as the mainstay of their diets (see table 1 on page 5).

Sugar, which has largely replaced these foods, is completely digested and leaves no fiber in the gut at all. Of course, we haven't only increased our consumption of sugar over the years. Our beef consumption has also vastly increased. But beef has as much fiber in it as ice cream: none whatsoever.

What you need are foods that provide bulk in the lower intestine, foods high in cellulose and other fibers that are not used by the body but passed through the intestinal tract to be eliminated after the nutrients have been extracted. Chewy, juicy, tough *plant* foods are generally high in roughage. Take note that the key word here is *plant* foods. Meats can also be described as chewy or tough, but as animal products, they have no fiber. *Only foods of plant origin contain fiber*.

Unprocessed wheat bran, which is produced by

the ton in the process of refining flour, may well be the best source of dietary fiber around. A few spoonfuls of bran added to your food each day will insure softer, bulkier stools for the constipation sufferer.

One British doctor who deserves much of the credit for the "discovery" that bran, as an exceptionally rich source of food fiber, is the best and most natural way to prevent and cure constipation, is Surgeon Captain Thomas Cleave of the Royal Navy.

As early as 1941, while he was senior medical officer on the battleship *King George V*, he began to report in the medical literature on the value of bran. Reviewing some of his past experiences, Captain Cleave relates that while he was serving on the battleship, there was a scarcity of fresh fruit and vegetables and he "found such bran invaluable for correcting the constipation (of) the ship's company . . . The sailors loved this stuff by comparison with purgatives . . . I think it is a great tragedy of our present age that, with Medical Research Council workers showing at least 15 percent of the population to be on regular purgatives, this precious material is ever lost through the manufacture of white flour."[3]

In addition to taking some bran each day, to guard against constipation increase your consumption of water. Most of us drink far too little. Much of the water you drink is absorbed in the small intestine, but of that which enters the large intestine, 80 percent is absorbed before the stool is passed. If you don't consume enough fluid to keep the colonic contents in a semiliquid form, the absorption of water from it will leave a stool that is hard, dry, and difficult to pass. If you have ever gone a long time without water or worked under conditions that caused you to perspire heavily, you may recall that your stool over the next day or two was drier and harder to pass than usual. The same thing happens when you neglect to drink enough fluid.

How much fluid is enough? At least six to eight glasses of water a day, over and above the liquids you normally consume with meals. This amounts to well over a quart of liquid daily; some doctors recommend at least two quarts each day.

If you have trouble getting down six to eight glasses of water a day, it will become much easier if you establish a pattern. Try placing six to eight pennies on the windowsill or counter by the kitchen sink. Each time you drink a glass of water, transfer a penny from one side of the sill or counter to the other. Continue to do this until you have moved all the pennies during the course of one day. If you're away from home for most of the day, you might want to carry with you a small notepad to mark down the glasses of water you drink.

Whether or not you are supplementing your diet with bran, you should always try to eat as many high-fiber foods as possible and cut down on fiberless, empty-calorie foods. And don't think sticking with high-fiber foods means a boring diet! Here are some examples of the good things you'll be able to enjoy.

As we learned in the last chapter, many fruit contain lots of bulk. If you can get them unsprayed, be sure to eat the skin, too. Or try your favorite fruit stewed or dried. The average person eats little or no fruit, except perhaps during the summer. But it is during the colder months when the diet is heavy and consists mostly of starches and protein, that fruit are needed most. And don't forget fresh vegetables—they are just as necessary.

Whole grain foods such as bulgur wheat, brown

rice, oatmeal, and buckwheat are other fine sources of roughage. In addition, they contain vitamins that are necessary for normal intestinal function. A simple change like switching from white bread to whole wheat bread will go a long way toward helping your lazy bowels to get moving again.

Untoasted peanuts, cashews, walnuts, filberts, almonds, and other nuts, as well as raw seeds—pumpkin, sunflower, and sesame—will also help restore your regularity. Dried beans are also good.

Another way to insure the prompt removal of food wastes from your body is bulk in the form of a daily green salad. In the springtime, earlier generations turned to dandelion, poke salad, mustard greens, and any number of wild plants to "cleanse the winter body." Any of the sturdy greens makes a welcome addition to the usual diet. For variety try chicory, romaine, curly endive, raw spinach, Chinese cabbage, and celery.

Now that you know more about how constipation comes about and the kinds of diseases it can lead to, perhaps you can better appreciate our need to regularly eliminate waste products. If you put a little bran in your diet each day, drink lots of water, and eat more roughage-rich foods, you should never need to worry about constipation again.

BRAN HELPS DIARRHEA, TOO

Contradictory as it may sound, bran can relieve diarrhea every bit as effectively as it alleviates constipation. The reason is that bran is a *normalizer* of bowel function, not simply a laxative. The absorptive and bulk-forming properties of bran that help form the large, soft stools which spell relief for constipation sufferers also help to "bind up" the watery stools of diarrhea.

Any bout with diarrhea, even if it lasts only a matter of hours, depletes the body of needed nourishment. The foods you eat simply slide through your intestines, scarcely staying in the intestinal tract long enough for any nutrients to be extracted. As far as nourishment is concerned, it's almost as if you didn't eat anything.

Foods rich in unrefined carbohydrates, pectin, or fiber, such as bran, help put an end to simple cases of diarrhea by providing bulk to slow the passage of food through the bowels.

Probably the first advocate of bran as a bowel normalizer was Sylvester Graham, for whom graham crackers and graham flour were named. In the nineteenth century, when the roller mill was first coming into wide use, Graham campaigned vigorously against the removal of bran and germ from grains in the refining of flour. His observations of the effectiveness of whole grains in relieving diarrhea as well as constipation anticipated by more than a century the evidence recently uncovered by British doctors of this double action of whole grains.

Documented clinical evidence of bran's effect on diarrhea came at last in 1972, in a study performed by Dr. Neil S. Painter and two colleagues, all associated with London's Manor House Hospital.[4] The doctors found in the course of their work with bran and patients suffering diverticular disease that bran relieved diarrhea, even in chronic cases. One unfortunate individual who needed to visit the bathroom

12 times a day, and another who did so 6 times a day, had only two bowel movements a day when their diets were supplemented with bran. Other investigations have reported this same result: bran is a natural regulator of bowel function.

Those people who find their system cannot tolerate bran as a diarrhea fighter may find success with either carob products or bananas. Both these foods contain sizeable amounts of pectin, which we noted before has a binding quality. Pectin swells in the digestive tract to help hold foods in the intestines and allow absorption of nutrients to take place. Bananas, in addition to providing pectin, also offer magnesium and potassium to help replace the minerals lost in diarrhea.

Of course, if your diarrhea is frequent and severe, by all means see a doctor. If the diarrhea involves a malabsorption syndrome, there may be a long-standing vitamin or mineral deficiency which will have to be corrected. Remember that during a siege of diarrhea, your body has no chance to absorb nutrients from food as it races through your intestinal tract. If the diarrhea is severe enough, it may be impossible to bring vitamin and mineral levels up to normal with the usual simple forms of supplementation—adjustments in diet or vitamin and mineral pills.

But for those occasional episodes when a virus or too-rich food loosens your bowels, bran could be just what the doctor ordered.

Constipation, Varicose
Veins, and
4 | # Hemorrhoids

Relieving constipation can mean freedom from the inevitability of many other painful and potentially dangerous disorders. Constipation with its attendant straining at stool has been found, for example, to be closely related to varicose veins (enlargement of the large veins in the legs) and femoral thrombosis (clotting in the large blood vessels in the thighs).

Varicose veins are among our most common venous disorders. They are unsightly and painful, they can in some cases become crippling, and there's really no reason we should ever get them! The reasons generally given for varicose veins are pregnancy, standing upright for long periods of time, and hereditary defects. But people in many other societies, the Masai tribes in Africa and the Maoris in New Zealand, for example, stand far longer than we do (they don't drive cars or work at desks) and have more children, and they never get varicose veins. Those painful, swollen veins peculiar to our advanced society cannot be fully explained by the conventionally accepted reasons.

Thrombosis in the femoral vein can be fatal if the clot breaks loose from the vein in the leg and travels through the bloodstream to lodge in the heart or lungs. Thrombosis is especially dangerous to postoperative patients, yet more and more of them have been developing blood clots in recent years. Doctors associate the higher incidence of thrombosis with the current lack of attention to the bowels before surgery. Preoperative patients are no longer routinely given enemas, with the result that the bowel becomes clogged and presses on the pelvic veins to cause clots.

What part does constipation play in the onset of varicose veins? Faulty elimination can cause varicose veins in two ways. First of all, constipation overloads the colon with wastes and causes the colon to press on the major veins in the pelvis, which carry blood back to the heart from veins in the legs and rectum. The pressure results in poor circulation to the veins of the legs and can be counted on to cause varicose veins or femoral thrombosis.

The second way in which constipation causes varicose veins is explained this way by researchers: When intestinal muscles must contract more violently to expel the small, hard stools of constipation, the increased pressure created in the colon is transmitted down through the pelvic veins, into the major veins of the legs. Since man has chosen to stand upright instead of on all fours, the blood in his legs must fight gravity in order to return to the heart for purification. An ingenious "muscle pump" enables the leg muscles to reinforce the pumping action of the heart to help push returning blood up the legs. In between pumps, a series of valves close to keep the blood from flowing back down the legs. The intense pressure transmitted to the leg veins by straining can cause these valves to malfunction and allow a backflow of blood to the legs, making the veins swollen and distended.

Our use of toilets also encourages varicose veins by the artificial position it forces our bodies to adopt to pass stool. People who live without the "conveniences" of Western civilization squat at stool; the squatting position blocks off the veins in the legs, and the straining and pushing caused by constipation exerts alarming amounts of pressure on these veins. Sitting on a toilet gives the veins in our legs no protection from the pressure—small wonder the valves in our legs may eventually give way!

There is a simple way to avoid all these problems and that is, of course, to avoid constipation. Clinical research being conducted in England shows that when food fiber in the form of bran is added to the diets of patients about to undergo surgery, the bowels don't clog with waste matter and don't press on the veins in the pelvis, and almost nobody develops femoral thrombosis after surgery.

Varicose veins aren't always caused by constipation. They can also be caused by obesity. Weighing significantly more than you should puts an unnatural strain on your legs, your circulatory system, and in fact, your whole body.

If we are to guard against venous problems, we must look to what we put into our bodies as well as how efficiently we eliminate it. Putting fiber in your diet can help you reduce your caloric intake as well as get your bowels in motion. (Obesity is discussed in more detail in "How to Overcome Obesity and Defeat Diabetes.")

HELP FOR HEMORRHOIDS

Hemorrhoids, that most embarrassing of afflictions, is another form of varicose veins. Nobody likes to talk about hemorrhoids and lots of people joke about it, but to the patient, the subject of hemorrhoids is a painfully serious matter. And perhaps the most agonizing aspect of his illness is that chances are he brought it on himself, for by far the more common cause of this often painful condition in the rectum or anus is constipation. And most constipation comes about through poor eating habits and lack of exercise.

But before we go into the causes, prevention, and treatment of hemorrhoids, let's first get a picture of the anatomy of this very common ailment. Briefly, hemorrhoids is a condition of distended (or varicose) veins in the anal region. There's the external type (piles), where distended veins obtrude in the areas just outside the sphincter (ringlike muscle) that surrounds the anus. Distended veins within the sphincter are referred to as internal hemorrhoids.

The reason why these veins tend to distend or become varicose has to do with gravity and man's upright position. As you know in the case of varicose veins in the legs, the problem is that when veins carry blood back to the heart from a low position in the body, they have to fight gravity. If the blood doesn't move upward fast enough, the pressure of too much blood within the vein dilates the vessel.

Unlike veins in the legs, which at least have the help of valves to prevent backflow of blood, the veins of the anal region are valveless. This omission has been called "nature's mistake," or you might think of it as our penalty for deciding to stand on two legs instead of four; there is no special need for valves in animals' rectal veins where this region of the body stands as high as the heart itself.

For us, whether sitting or standing, it is obvious that gravity encourages venous blood to pool in the rectal region and cause distended veins. Two different types of pressure exerted from outside the vein can either worsen or better this condition.

The muscles around the rectum, by providing counter-pressure, should normally prevent distended veins. This mechanism is the same as that provided by healthy leg muscles in keeping the leg veins in order, or by elastic stockings, which by their own pressure counter the pressure in distended veins of the leg. However, bad posture and flabby abdominal muscles, caused by lack of exercise, allow your sphincter muscle to sag until it can no longer give support to your rectal veins.

The kind of pressure that worsens the varicose condition is that which obstructs the blood flow upward. Anything that pinches the vein or squeezes on it making it difficult for the blood to get through serves to increase internal pressure—and makes for distended vessels. For example, women are particularly vulnerable to hemorrhoids during pregnancy. As the enlarged uterus pushes aside abdominal organs, it is likely to pinch veins—those coming from the rectal area no less than the veins of the legs. An abdominal or rectal tumor will do the same thing—though in this case, of course, the resulting hemorrhoids are the least of your worries.

But undoubtedly the primary culprit in the manufacture of hemorrhoids is straining of the abdominal muscles—and the most common everyday practitioner of such straining is the constipated wretch sitting on the toilet in seclusion and despair. The pressure of straining to expel a small stool tightly constricts blood vessels in the rectal area.

Obviously, if you would avoid hemorrhoids you must avoid constipation. And, while some doleful victims of this condition may object that this is "easier said than done," it really is possible to change your way of life to eliminate this unhappy and widespread affliction of Western civilized man.

TREATING HEMORRHOIDS

Hemorrhoids are acutely and painfully evident to the victim when they are the external type (piles). The distended veins, often containing small blood clots, obtrude in the anal area outside the sphincter, and they are misery to sit on. Pain is sometimes relieved by minor office surgery whereby the clots are cut out.

Because within the sphincter there are far fewer sensory nerves, the internal type of hemorrhoids can be painless. You know that something is wrong if one of the swelled veins ruptures and you find bleeding from the rectum. Sometimes an internal hemorrhoid prolapses—that is, comes down through the sphincter and has to be pushed back up into the rectum. Internal hemorrhoids can obstruct bowel movement and cause excess secretion of mucus.

As in the case of constipation, for the treatment of hemorrhoids you should avoid the much advertised over-the-counter remedies. A few give temporary relief of discomfort and pain—but none has any lasting effect, and for temporary relief a sitz bath that you give yourself at home is probably as effective as anything you can purchase.

It is possible that hemorrhoids might be reduced by an adequate intake of vitamin E. We make this suggestion on the basis of Dr. Wilfrid E. Shute's success with alpha tocopherol (vitamin E) in reducing varicose veins in the legs. It seems at least highly possible that vitamin E therapy might also be effective in shrinking "varicose veins of the rectal area."

Furthermore, vitamin E's remarkable ability to prevent or dissolve blood clots, or thrombi, should make this vitamin an extremely helpful agent for eliminating the clots found so distressing in piles.

So try vitamin E, by all means. But, if you presently suffer from hemorrhoids, you shouldn't let any hope of self-treatment keep you from the doctor's. For, while hemorrhoids are usually caused by constipation, you cannot be sure that something more serious may not be responsible. As mentioned earlier, a tumor pressing against the vein can cause the vessel to distend. So an early checkup might be the occasion of spotting a cancer while it can still be checked. Liver ailment also can promote hemorrhoids by obstructing the return flow of blood from the anal veins.

Especially you should remember that if you have bleeding from the rectum you cannot assume that it is "merely" hemorrhoids. It could be cancer, ulcerative colitis, or other inflammations that require treatment. A visit to the doctor is a must.

In really advanced cases of hemorrhoids, surgical removal of the offending veins is the only answer for permanent relief. However, mild or beginning cases can often be reversed if the cause of the trouble is eliminated. Hemorrhoids brought on by pregnancy, for example, frequently shrink back to normal after delivery. And a similar reprieve often blesses the person who corrects his persistent constipation.

So, if constipation is your problem, you know what the answer is. The guidelines are all there, and now it's up to you. So get moving!

5 | Building a Healthy Heart

Heart disease is our number one killer. More Americans are dying each year of heart disease than any other illness. And sadly, many of these deaths are needless. They could have been prevented; not with sophisticated drugs but with some simple dietary modifications. Putting more fiber in your diet can guard your heart and circulatory system against the devastating effects of a "civilized" diet.

The relationship between cholesterol and heart disease has been at the center of a major medical debate for over 20 years. A basic understanding of the issues involved will help you to better comprehend the role of fiber in protecting your heart.

There are many ways in which the heart may become diseased—the heart muscle itself can weaken, the built-in electrical stimulator that keeps it going may become erratic, the lining of the heart can become infected, or a heart valve may become faulty. But the great killer among heart diseases in the United States and other Western societies is coronary heart disease—or "heart attack" as it is popularly known.

Its precursor is atherosclerosis, a disease in which hardened fatty plaques (composed largely of cholesterol) build up on the inside of artery walls. A coronary artery (one feeding the heart) may become completely occluded, or closed off, by plaque buildup. Or it may become so narrow and its once smooth inner walls so rough and jagged that a clot forms (coronary thrombosis) and plugs up the passage, preventing blood and oxygen from reaching the heart. That's the classic "heart attack."

Heart attacks and high serum cholesterol levels have been linked together statistically, both in epidemiological studies (in which an entire population or societal group is monitored) and in the study of individuals in the famous Framingham, Massachusetts, research project. In Framingham, after more than 20 years of regular medical checkups on more than 5,000 initially healthy men and women, it was determined that high levels of cholesterol in the blood serum do indeed mean an increased risk of death from heart attack. There is clear statistical association.

The medical establishment has adopted the position that this is a case of cause and effect and that bringing down cholesterol levels will lower the incidence of heart deaths. Unfortunately, singling out dietary cholesterol and saturated fats as the prime villains of the heart disease story has deprived many patients of such fine, nutritious (but cholesterol-rich) foods as eggs and liver. Patients are made to give up all fats derived from animals, such as butter, cheese, whole milk, and all but the leanest of meats.

But this kind of harsh dietary restriction isn't always necessary. Doctors have found that introducing more fiber into the diet lowers serum cholesterol in individuals with a high content of cholesterol in their blood (i.e., potential heart attack victims). Conversely, when fiber consumption is reduced, cholesterol levels rise.

WHERE DOES THE CHOLESTEROL GO?

The precise mechanism whereby dietary fiber might influence serum cholesterol is not yet fully understood. But possibly it is related to fiber's effect on bile acids. The larger the stools a person forms, the more bile acids he excretes, and a high-fiber diet helps insure these large stools.

But what have bile acids to do with this whole cholesterol picture?

Cholesterol (which we synthesize in our own bodies as well as ingest with foods) is the precursor of bile acids. From cholesterol in the liver, bile acids are manufactured and sent via the bile duct into the top portion of the small intestine (duodenum). Here their job is to help in the digestive breakdown of dietary fats, after which function some bile acids travel down the intestinal tract and are excreted with the feces, while the greater portion is reabsorbed into the body and travels back to the liver via the bloodstream.

You can see why a dietary factor that increases fecal excretion of bile acids might also lower serum cholesterol levels. For as long as plenty of reabsorbed bile acids are returning to the liver, there is no need to manufacture great quantities more, and cholesterol that would have been used for bile acid synthesis is not metabolized in this fashion but remains in the system. Thus, the major mechanism whereby cholesterol leaves the body—by catabolic metabolism into bile acids—is reduced in efficiency when our natural diet is deprived of its fiber content.

Moreover, there is evidence that high fiber content in the intestines also reduces the absorption of cholesterol taken in with foods. So a high-residue diet, typical of primitive societies, would promote the excretion of both the catabolized cholesterol (present as bile acids) and ingested cholesterol.

Of course we know that other factors beside fiber deficiency help cause coronary heart disease. There are such well-known and undisputed steps for reducing heart risk as: don't smoke, maintain ideal weight, exercise regularly. And when it comes to diet, we know that fiber deficiency cannot be the only culprit.

Hand in hand with fiber deficiency goes overconsumption of sugar. Researchers have found that adding sugar to the diet raises the level of blood cholesterol.

Just stop and think, for a moment, about the average American diet—maybe your own diet. Our systems are full of cholesterol because we're eating lots of sugar (the average American puts away more than 100 pounds of sugar in a year), but our meals contain so little fiber that much of that cholesterol isn't even being metabolized! Is it any wonder heart disease is our number one killer?

Perhaps you're already aware of the need to keep your sugar consumption to a minimum. Many heart patients are tuned in to the importance of a good diet, and many conscientiously try to cut out sweets, alcohol, and excess fat. But there is another dimension to diet which is of great importance to the heart patient, although few know much about it, and others prefer not to think about it.

We are talking about what happens to the food you eat—regardless of whether it is high or low in cholesterol—when it reaches your lower bowels and needs to be eliminated.

Many of us have heard of someone we knew who had a weak heart and was found dead in the bathroom. Depending on your age, you may also be aware that there is a strange tendency for people to collapse in the bathroom even when they are not known to have a bad heart.

The blunt truth is that the majority of these people have died before their time as an indirect result of one of the most common diseases in the modern world—constipation.

It is not constipation itself which poses the danger but straining at stool. The abnormal stress which straining puts on the heart is much greater than you might imagine. In fact, even people who have no signs of a heart problem can dangerously overburden their hearts when straining. Tests have shown in people with no previous history of heart disorder that straining produces significant changes in heart rate, blood pressure, and electrocardiograph patterns. Further, these changes closely resemble those which are observed in known heart patients.

Specifically, about 12 percent of straining episodes are found to be of sufficient intensity and duration to produce notable abnormalities. The frequency of such incidents is increased five times by the problem of constipation.

Another aspect of the problem involves the

changes in size undergone by the veins in the rectum and legs during bathroom straining. These changes are much greater in constipation and sometimes may cause blood clots to break loose from veins and travel toward the heart.

Paul M. Zoll, M.D., writing in the *Journal of the American Medical Association* (September 1961) points out that the marked increase in pressure within the entire thoracic and abdominal cavity while straining could cause a diverticulum of the bowel (which will be explained in "Ending the Misery of Irritable Colon and Diverticular Disease") or an aneurysm (blood-filled dilatation) of a major blood vessel or of the heart itself to rupture. Straining can also bring an angina or "prolonged cardiac pain in a patient with extensive coronary disease," he warns.

So while constipation certainly isn't fun for anybody, it can be downright dangerous and life threatening to older people and those of any age who are in a weakened condition. People who are confined to bed following surgery or hospitalization are particularly vulnerable—not only to constipation but to the damage which straining or fecal impaction can cause.

Once again, the right kind of diet could be your salvation. If you have heart trouble (and to be on the safe side even if you don't), cut down on the amount of sweet foods you consume. Cutting out sweets can also protect you from obesity and diabetes, as we'll see in "How To Overcome Obesity and Defeat Diabetes." So, keep your cholesterol down, your fiber level up, and make constipation a thing of the past.

How To Overcome
Obesity and Defeat
6 Diabetes

Overweight is the most common form of malnutrition in the United States today—as many as 30 percent of young men and 20 percent of young women weigh too much. More than half the population over the age of 40 is too heavy. And this happens despite the fact that many fat people are constantly trying to reduce and despite high costs of food and worldwide shortages.

The overweight syndrome hardly exists at all, though, in many underdeveloped countries, even those with ample supplies of food. People there eat what they want, yet stay trim all their lives. True, there are some fat people in any society, but they are rare in places where people live on simple, rustic, fiber-rich food. Just think how nice it would be to eat as much as you wanted and still stay thin!

Many medical experts are convinced that obesity is not always the result of eating too much food. It can just as easily be caused by eating the wrong kinds of food, which prevent our digestive system from functioning as it should. This theory makes a good deal of sense. Consider these circumstances:

The purpose of the gastrointestinal tract is to process food and extract from it the nutrients the body needs. A multitude of complex operations all fit smoothly together to perform these two functions. But suppose the food presented to the gastrointestinal tract was already processed and extracted before it was eaten. When the food industry does the job the gastrointestinal tract was meant to do, what happens to that finely tuned digestive system? It seems only reasonable to assume its function will be in some way disturbed, and the rest of the body will be affected.

Suppose we compare the function of the digestive system to the operation of an iron ore smelting works.[1] Normally, the works is supplied with crude iron ore which it must process and from which it extracts the iron. If one day the suppliers begin to send pure iron in place of a portion of the usual crude ore, two things may be expected to happen.

First, the extra amount of pure iron will cause a stockpile to build up unless special efforts are made to get rid of the excess. Second, since less ore now needs to be processed, part of the plant will shut down, and workers will be laid off. The unemployed workers will be discontent and will probably start disputes and even strikes.

Supplying the human digestive system with processed foods causes the same two problems—stockpiling and unemployment with its subsequent negative effects.

As carbohydrate is the nutrient whose properties are most altered by the refining process (protein and fat are relatively unchanged; vitamins and minerals provide no calories), we will focus our attention on this nutrient.

The major role of carbohydrate is to provide energy for the body. It also enables the body to manufacture some of the vitamin B complex. The human race, considered as a whole, gets 70 percent of its energy from carbohydrates. Starch, glucose, sucrose, and lactose are the most familiar of the carbohydrates. Starch is the form in which plants store energy for future use; it is found in seeds (grains), legumes, and roots (potatoes). In our bodies, digestion breaks down starch into glucose, which can be used for energy. Extra glucose is converted to fat and stored in body tissues.

White sugar is the most concentrated of all refined carbohydrate foods and as such poses the biggest threat to the digestive system.

OBESITY COMES FROM STOCKPILING ENERGY

Obesity is generally defined as exceeding your ideal weight by ten percent or more. Actually though, going above your ideal weight by any amount constitutes overweight, which means that even the astounding assessment of the number of obese adults in this country is too low. Think of all the people you know who are only five or ten pounds overweight—not a full ten percent but overweight none the less.

The great proportion of too-heavy people in our culture means that Western man has a hard time keeping his energy intake in balance with his energy output. It seems he does not *choose* to be fat, for overweight is known to be related to a number of serious diseases, and it certainly is not considered stylish.

Probably the most rational explanation for all this excess weight is that we are overnourished by the refined carbohydrates so abundant in our food.

The primary sources of carbohydrates in today's typical Western diet are white flour and white sugar—two heavily refined foods. White flour has had most of its fiber removed, and sugar has lost absolutely all of its bulk. These foods supply energy (calories) without the fiber that should go along to make us feel full. Starches and sugars are never found in their natural state without fiber (with the single exception of honey, which has really been processed by bees). When we eat carbohydrates as they occur in nature, with fiber intact, we become full before we take in too many calories. But when we eat fiber-depleted carbohydrate foods, like sugar, we don't feel satisfied until long after we've taken in the amount of calories we need.

HOW REFINED FOODS HARM OUR BODIES

Fiberless foods cause several unhealthy changes in our gastrointestinal tract and help to create problems in addition to stockpiling energy. For one thing, less gastric juice is secreted to digest these foods, so the digesting food doesn't take up much space in our stomachs and we don't feel full. We are encouraged to overeat.

Also, sugar holds food in the stomach for an abnormally long time (white flour does too, although to a somewhat lesser degree). This stasis is believed to occur because when the stomach is less distended, it is less stimulated to contract, and food does not move on down the gastrointestinal tract as promptly as it should. Many researchers have become convinced that food remaining too long in the stomach is a cause of dyspepsia (indigestion) and heartburn and may also influence the development of peptic ulcers. In addition, the stomach contents are more acid after a meal of refined food than after fibrous foods are consumed. (A more detailed explanation of stomach problems appears in "Fiber Helps Your Stomach, Too.")

As we have discussed earlier, intestinal transit times are markedly slower when refined foods are eaten. Thus, there is a greater chance for nutrients (and energy) to be absorbed from food as it passes through the intestine.

As can be expected, foods with all their fiber intact have an opposite effect on the digestive system than refined foods. Experiments have shown that increasing fiber intake causes more carbohydrates to be excreted along with food wastes.

In a study performed in San Francisco in 1972, 13 men already on a low-cholesterol diet were told to reduce their intake of carbohydrates, especially sugar. The low-carbohydrate diet supplied the same amount of calories as did the previous one, but the men lost weight at an average rate of four pounds in six months.[2]

The wealth of evidence like that above shows that our mass obesity problem is not the result of overeating but of *getting too much out of our food*. This unhappy situation occurs because we satisfy a normal appetite with refined carbohydrate foods that supply us with too much energy in relation to satiety.

If this theory is correct, *unrefined* carbohydrates should not be fattening, and indeed, statistics show that members of societies in which large amounts of such foods (unrefined grains, cornmeal, beans, etc.) are eaten each day are almost never overweight.

WHY SUGAR DESERVES THE BLAME

Although many of the carbohydrate foods we eat today are refined—white rice, packaged cereals, instant potatoes—the most abundant and at the same time most harmful are white flour and white sugar. Sugar is without a doubt the greater of the two evils, and here's why. First of all, sugar is simply more refined. Sugar represents only 16 percent of the sugar beet, making it a vastly more concentrated product than white flour, which is 70 percent of the original wheat berry. In order to eat enough sweet foods to satisfy your hunger, you must take in enormous amounts of calories—far, far too many for your body's needs.

Sound hard to believe? Try this test: put a tea-spoonful of sugar in your mouth and let it dissolve. Now ask yourself honestly if you feel as if you've eaten anything, if you feel any fuller. The truthful answer to both these questions should be "no." What has happened is that without any chewing, with only the slightest movement of your tongue, you have soaked up 16 calories in a few seconds. You can imagine how many calories you'd consume if you filled up on sugar, yet if you depend on heavily refined foods to fill a major portion of your dietary needs, you are in all likelihood doing that very thing. All those extra calories don't just float around inside your body— they are converted into fat and go right to the tissues to be stored in the form of a potbelly, double chin, or bulgy thighs.

A second strike against sugar is that while bread consumption has fallen, obesity is ever on the rise. These circumstances further shift the heaviest blame away from white flour. As our bread consumption drops, our intake of sweets continues to increase. A stroll through any supermarket will show you aisles and aisles crowded with sodas, ice cream, cookies, pudding mixes, sugary snacks, instant beverage mixes, and candy.

If you take a closer look at the candy section, you'll find that it's getting harder all the time to buy a single candy bar. Most of it is sold in multipacks or eight-ounce family-size bars. One of those family-size bars provides more than 1,280 calories! You'd have to eat 32 slices of bread to get that many calories, but that's the kind of food America is snacking on.

There's even more evidence to convict sugar of making us fat. Sugar can be (and is) drunk in many beverages; flour cannot. Finally, sugar is so *available*. It's all around us, in vending machines, convenience foods, even breakfast foods. You munch on sweets in many places where nutritious food is nowhere to be seen: at the ball park, the movies, the corner newsstand, bus terminals, gas stations, laundromats, even college dormitories! Think of all the places where you'll find a soda machine but can't get a drink of plain old water!

In nature, sugar is simply not this easy to get at. It is only found as a component of a whole food, not by itself. The refining process has made available to us much, much more sugar than we could possibly get on our own from whole foods.

BRAN CUTS CALORIE ABSORPTION

Take heart—none of us has to drown in this sea of sugar. Bran can be the answer to a weight watcher's prayer. Increasing the amount of fiber in your diet can cut the caloric value of foods, even sugary foods, to help you lose weight without starving yourself, and bran is the easiest form of fiber to use.

Dr. Kenneth Heaton of Bristol University in England points out that food fiber hinders energy or calorie intake.[3] When ten young women were fed diets of increasing fiber content, their waste matter contained progressively more calories, fat, and protein. The calories absorbed fell from 97 percent on a low-residue diet to 92.5 percent on a high-fiber diet. Volunteers eating bread diets excreted 321 calories a day on whole meal bread but only 99 calories a day on white bread. Since this difference is considerably more than can be accounted for simply by the presence of undigested fiber in the stools, these studies indicate that fiber hinders intestinal absorption. No one is quite sure how it works. But Dr. Heaton postulates that fiber cells may simply act as a mechanical barrier which impedes the passage of digestive enzymes and keeps some of the digestive nutrients from coming in contact with the absorptive membrane of the intestinal wall.

Food fiber provides other obstacles to energy intake. A given amount of a fiber-containing food, such as whole wheat flour, supplies fewer calories than an equal amount of the same food in refined form, in this case white flour, because the fiber takes up space that is occupied by nutrients in the refined product (see Appendix B).

Fiber requires vigorous chewing which slows down intake. Chewing also limits the amount of food which can be consumed, because it promotes the secretion of saliva and gastric juices which distend the stomach. Further, indigestible food fiber takes up space in the stomach and bowel. The same amount of sugar contained in one candy bar is found naturally in three pounds of apples. It's easy to eat the calories in the form of the candy bar, but how many people could eat three pounds of apples at a sitting?

DIABETES AND REFINED CARBOHYDRATES

Diabetes and obesity are closely related—many diabetics are overweight and many heavy people, whether they know it or not, are diabetics. For this reason, obesity has long been thought to be a cause of diabetes. Now, however, obesity is believed to develop under the same conditions as diabetes, but not to cause it.

Surgeon Captain Cleave, the man who first treated the constipation of British sailors with bran, has said for many years that diabetes is brought on by overconsumption of refined, fiberless foods, particularly sugar.[4] Now at last the rest of the medical world is starting to listen. The concentrated carbohydrates contained in such foods place a strain on the insulin-producing mechanism of the pancreas. The progression toward diabetes is gradual—it may take as long as 20 years until the disease actually appears.

The quantity of food energy hitting the pancreas is not the only factor in determining when diabetes will strike; the rate at which the energy is delivered also plays an important role. The Irish, for example, used to live mostly on potatoes, a high-carbohydrate food, but they seldom got diabetes. Of course, we must consider that when people work harder, they use up more energy and so need to consume more carbohydrates. Our sedentary life-style means we need a smaller amount of carbohydrates than do members of more active societies. But the fact that carbohydrates in their natural, unrefined form have never been associated with diabetes points to refined, concentrated carbohydrates as the primary cause of the disease.

When refined carbohydrate foods such as sugar are eaten, energy hits the pancreas at a rapid pace, because the carbohydrates in such foods are densely concentrated.

Like the rest of the diseases of civilization, diabetes is not found among people who rely on unrefined foods for their carbohydrates. Also, during World War II, when rationing made white flour and sugar scarce, the incidence of diabetes dropped. In England, deaths from diabetes dropped by more than 50 percent during this period.

On the other hand, people who switch from unprocessed foods to refined foods develop more diabetes. In Rhodesia, for example, city dwellers are consuming a more Westernized diet, and their rate of diabetes is increasing in direct proportion.[5]

It will probably come as no surprise that doctors are finally beginning to recognize the ability of a high-fiber diet to control diabetes. Dr. Cleave recommends returning to whole, unrefined foods to obtain carbohydrates in their original, unconcentrated form. That means cutting out sugar wherever possible. And of course, bran will also help keep you from overloading your pancreas with energy.

HOW GALLSTONES ARE RELATED

Doctors have noted that many patients suffering bowel problems also have trouble with their gallbladders. The available evidence suggests that the same refined diet that causes bowel disease, obesity, and diabetes is also responsible for gallstones. Dr. Christopher D. Holland documented the number of gallbladder operations performed in the Bristol, England area since 1933. He found that from the 1930s to the 1950s, the rate hovered around 30 cases per 100,000 persons, then suddenly leaped to over 75 cases per 100,000.[6]

Not only is gallbladder surgery on the rise, but the disease is beginning to attack growing numbers of younger people and people among whom it was formerly rare, such as Canadian Eskimos and the Japanese. As gallbladder disease spreads, more attention is being given to pinpointing the factors responsible for its development.

Gallstones which form from extra cholesterol in the bloodstream are common among people eating a refined diet but are practically unheard of in primitive cultures. Experiments involving both people and animals have now shown that a deficiency of fiber and an excess of sugar interfere with the functions of bile and cholesterol and allow a buildup of cholesterol in the bloodstream.

The amount of cholesterol in the blood (called the serum cholesterol level) is determined not only by the quantity ingested in food, but also by how much the body 1) manufactures, 2) changes into bile acids, 3) returns from the bowel back to the liver via the bloodstream, and 4) expels in waste matter. Unless all these factors are balanced, cholesterol can accumulate in the blood, where it may lead to a number of circulatory disorders or gallstones.

Medical researchers have found that animals and people on high-fiber diets excrete more cholesterol and more bile acids (which are used by the liver in the manufacture of cholesterol) than those on refined diets, thereby lowering the level of serum cholesterol.

Dr. Heaton observed that plasma triglyceride levels fell markedly in 17 subjects given bran for five weeks. The drop was especially striking in subjects who had exceedingly high levels to begin with.[7] The plasma triglyceride level is related to the amount of cholesterol in the blood because it correlates closely with the rate at which the liver synthesizes cholesterol. A fall in the triglyceride level indicates that the liver is manufacturing less cholesterol, so there will be less cholesterol released into the blood. Thus, the chances that gallstones will form are considerably fewer.

7 | Fiber Helps Your Stomach, Too

As we have seen, irregularities in bowel function caused by a highly refined diet can also effect the circulatory system and encourage obesity and diabetes. But the chemistry of the bowels is complex, and we must not lose sight of the fact that they do not function alone but are part of the gastrointestinal tract, which also includes the stomach. Therefore, we might expect that fiber deficiency causes problems in the stomach as well as in the bowels, and indeed it does.

If you remember from chapter 6, fiberless food remains in the stomach for inordinately long periods of time. This stasis occurs because refined food does not fully distend the stomach, and when the stomach is not distended, it does not contract to push its contents toward the bowels. Many medical researchers believe that digested food staying too long in the stomach is responsible for many cases of indigestion and heartburn.

These very symptoms were found to be relieved by a high-fiber, low-sugar diet. Dr. Neil S. Painter, whose landmark work with bran and diverticular disease will be discussed in the next chapter, found that the diet his patients were following to relieve diverticular symptoms also got rid of nausea and heartburn! These ailments are not generally associated with illness of the lower bowel, but their disappearance indicates that a high-fiber diet is important to the well-being of the entire gastrointestinal tract not just the lower bowel. The debilitating effects of a refined diet go far beyond simple constipation, and even beyond occasional heartburn and indigestion. More serious stomach disorders are now being blamed on refined foods. One of these is peptic ulcer; another is hiatus hernia, both common diseases in Western societies.

The same stasis of food responsible for heartburn also plays a role in the development of peptic ulcer. Peptic ulcer occurs when stomach acids attack the lining of the stomach walls and cause an open sore. Acid coming in contact with the sore causes intense pain. When digested food is held in the stomach, acid is held there too, and the prolonged contact with the stomach walls increases the chances for ulceration to occur. Also, stomach contents are more acid after refined foods are digested than after a meal of fibrous foods. Adequate dietary fiber is necessary, then, to protect our stomachs from the conditions which could allow ulcers to develop.

Refining eliminates from some foods another important form of protection for the stomach—protein. When wheat is processed into white flour, a substantial amount of its protein is lost. The protein is needed to act as a buffer against the hydrochloric acid in the stomach, helping to protect the stomach walls from the acid attacks that could lead to ulcers. The absence of so much of this protein therefore weakens the stomach's defenses against ulcers.

HIATUS HERNIA

A more serious stomach problem is hiatus hernia. This disorder is becoming increasingly more common, and Dr. Denis Burkitt and his colleague, Dr. Peter A. James, have theorized that it is also caused by insufficient roughage.[1] Hiatus hernia is a protrusion of the stomach upward through the wall of the diaphragm. Drs. Burkitt and James believe that the abnormally high pressures in the abdomen which are caused by straining at stool play an important part in the development of hiatus hernia.

As evidence they cite the fact that the incidence of hiatus hernia in Western countries has climbed sharply since World War II, and although detection methods have improved, that alone is not enough to explain the tremendous increase in the number of cases. Developing countries do not match the high incidence rates of the West, a fact that indicates the causes are environmental rather than genetic.

The previously accepted explanations of what causes hiatus hernia are no longer acceptable. Drs. Burkitt and James state that intense abdominal pressures are *not* produced by

1) tumors—abdominal tumors get much larger in countries where surgical treatment is not available, and these countries have low rates of hiatus hernia;

2) pregnancy—women in countries with low hernia rates are pregnant far more often than women living in high-incidence countries;

3) obesity—the relationship between obesity and hiatus hernia seems to be one of common cause rather than of cause and effect;

4) constricting clothes—if clothes are the cause of hernia, in light of changes in clothing styles, the hernia rate should have fallen, instead of rising, over the past 20 years.

If all of the old explanations for hiatus hernia are discarded, we are left with faulty diet as the prime suspect The high intracolonic pressures needed to expel the small, hard stools resulting from a refined diet are now being blamed for hiatus hernia as well as other ailments. The pressure of straining, unlike pressure produced by a cough, can be sustained for several seconds. Eventually, the stomach is pushed through the diaphragm wall at its weakest point.

Hiatus hernia doesn't always produce symptoms, but often it is accompanied by pains in the upper abdomen. The condition is common, and its prevalence increases with age. In fact, hiatus hernia is demonstrable in nearly half the population of the Western world over the age of 50.[2] The fact that the geographic distribution of hiatus hernia so closely parallels the distribution of diverticulitis and the rest of the diseases of civilization indicates that it stems from the same basic problem: lack of fiber in the diet.

Ending The Misery of Irritable Colon and Diverticular Disease

8

If you are past the age of 40 and have all your life been eating a standard American diet overloaded with refined carbohydrate foods, there is a 50 percent chance that you will eventually experience the pain and distress of diverticular disease of the colon. It may begin with persistent constipation, sometimes alternating with diarrhea, and soon involve nausea, vomiting, abdominal swelling, cramps and pain in your lower left side. Should you try to ignore these discomforts, chills and fever will add to the general feeling of sickness.

Diverticular disease in its mildest form will provoke occasional tenderness or cramping; if your case is more severe, the pain and inflammation can grow so intense that the diseased portion of your colon will have to be removed surgically. If your condition continues to worsen, complications may develop, affecting the bladder, small intestine, and uterus. Hemorrhage and rectal bleeding may ensue and in extreme cases the result is death.

The basic lesion in diverticular disease is the diverticulum, a pea-sized balloon poking through the muscular lining of the lower bowel. Actually, it is not so much the diverticula themselves that cause trouble but the inflammation which occurs when food particles become lodged in these little sacs, often along with bacteria. Then the condition is known as diverticulitis.

How are these evil little herniations formed in the first place?

Intestinal walls are made up of two sets of muscles: a longitudinal set that come together at the rectum, and a series of circular muscles that wrap around the entire length of the intestine's inner wall. Waste matter is normally moved through the sacs of the lower gut by waves of muscular contraction. When the bowels are relatively full of waste matter, as they are in vegetarians, for example, or people in underdeveloped countries who eat a diet high in roughage, the muscles surrounding the intestines need to contract only slightly to move it along. But when waste matter is scanty and compacted, as it is in those eating a soft or highly refined diet, the muscles have to contract with much greater force to create the pressure required to keep things moving.

It's something like squeezing a tube of toothpaste; when the tube is full or nearly full, you only have to press lightly on the tube to expel the toothpaste. But when the tube is nearly empty, you have to squeeze and squeeze to get it out. When the intestines contain only scanty waste matter, they must contract to the point where they form individual bladders, or segments, closed on one end and open on the other, in order to empty themselves.

It is these powerful contractions that are the source of much misery. The most intense contractions take place in the sigmoid colon, which is the S-shaped portion of the colon leading directly to the rectum, and which is quite narrow but lined with powerful muscles. Tremendous pressure builds up under these contractions, and because the human bowel was never designed to handle such pressure, the all-too-frequent result is that the bowel lining bursts through the surrounding muscles and forms a balloon or diverticulum. Some people have a great many of these diverticula, particularly in the sigmoid colon.

For many years, it was the general medical practice to prescribe a low-residue, soft, bland diet for people with diverticular problems. This treatment was largely based on the observation that foods with roughage sometimes caused irritation of the bowels, and when whole seeds were swallowed without being chewed, they sometimes lodged in the sacs. Now, however, doctors are beginning to recognize the advantages of a high-roughage diet, which eliminates the dangerous intracolonic pressures created by intense contractions of the colon muscles.

FROM SPASTIC COLON TO DIVERTICULITIS

Most of us have heard at sometime or other of an ailment known as spastic colon, or the irritable bowel syndrome. Both these terms refer to a common set of symptoms including constipation and irregularity, colicky pains in the lower abdomen, and a general feeling of just plain discomfort in the abdominal area.

Few people get really upset about irritable bowel syndrome—it is usually shrugged off as an inevitable consequence of middle age. But this chronic state of irritation is now believed to be the forerunner of diverticulosis, which cannot be cured once it is acquired.

Diverticulosis is the name given to the presence of the tiny balloons, or diverticula, along the colon walls, whether or not painful symptoms are present (there is usually little pain when the diverticula are not inflamed).

Diverticulitis, as the name implies, is the inflammation of the diverticula, and it causes extreme pain. Inflammation occurs when waste matter collects in these pockets and ferments there for long periods of time. Bits of undigested food, such as bone chips, may lodge there and cause the painful inflammation.

In most cases, the first attack of diverticulitis is a warning that a second and more severe attack is on its way. If the attacks continue, surgery will eventually be necessary.

Diverticular disease in all its forms is the most common bowel affliction in the Western world today. Studies from the United States, Britain, Australia, and France have revealed that between one-third and one-half of the people more than 40 years of age in those countries have diverticula, or abnormal outgrowths of the intestinal wall. As these people get older, their susceptibility to the condition increases so much that the disease strikes two-thirds of those civilized people who have reached the age of 80.

Yet, diverticular disease was practically unknown before the twentieth century. It was identified over a hundred years ago, but the condition was so seldom seen that it wasn't even mentioned in medical textbooks until after 1920. Within 70 years, the average human life span, diverticulitis has become a major health problem!

Recent evidence points to the food we eat as the factor responsible for catapulting diverticular disease from obscurity into the medical spotlight. In fact, two of the foremost authorities in the field believe that the only way to "contract" diverticular disease is to eat your way into it.

A VEGETABLE FIBER DEFICIENCY DISEASE

Dr. Neil S. Painter, senior surgeon at Manor House Hospital in London, whose previous studies of diverticular disease have contributed to new methods of treating the disorder, and Dr. Denis P. Burkitt, noted British medical researcher whose foresight while working in Africa led to the discovery of the cause of an African lymph gland cancer now known as Burkitt's lymphoma (his work was discussed in chapter 1), have stated that "diverticulosis appears to be a deficiency disease caused by the refining of carbohydrates which entails the removal of vegetable fiber from the diet. Consequently," they add, "we consider it to be preventable."[1] In other words, if a diet of natural, whole foods instead of highly refined products was eaten in Western cultures, diverticular disease could disappear.

The reason, they say, is that a refined carbohydrate diet devoid of roughage after a long period of time is responsible for narrowing of the colon, which in turn invites inefficient segmentation and the formation of diverticula. On the other hand, an unrefined diet containing plenty of roughage keeps the diameter of the colon wide and functioning normally.

The foundation for much of the investigation into

fiber and the colon was laid in East Africa, where Dr. Burkitt spent 20 years. He found that in rural areas of Africa where Western civilization has not intruded the disease is almost never seen by doctors.

Drs. Painter and Burkitt commented that their survey of worldwide reports "confirms that diverticular disease is rarely found in people whose eating habits changed but little up to the present."[2]

In his 20 years of practicing surgery in Africa, Dr. Burkitt did not encounter a single case of diverticulitis. The rural Africans had none of the so-called diseases of civilization. They had no bowel cancer, no obesity, no diabetes, and no hernias.

As we learned in chapter 1, this is not a matter of geography, because Africans who live in cities and eat Westernized diets soon develop the same bowel problems that plague the Englishmen who live in these cities and who eat a strictly Western diet.

Why? Because the rural African eats a diet which contains large amounts of indigestible roughage, or fiber. His grain is refined only slightly, by hand, and thus retains much of the bran which is missing completely from the white flour we consume. He eats a great deal of fruit, vegetables, seeds, and roots, all of which are also full of fiber. All of this indigestible matter is a positive blessing to his lower intestine. In addition, Dr. Burkitt believes that the absence of refined sugar from the diet of these rural Africans is another important plus factor in maintaining the amazing health of their lower digestive systems.

When you visit your doctor to seek relief from your bowel troubles, assuming he diagnoses your problem correctly, he will recommend either surgery or the dietary regimen still generally accepted by the medical profession as correct for diverticulitis of the colon. As described by the *Merck Manual,* a physician's reference book, diverticulitis calls for a low-residue diet, one meant "to spare an inflamed or irritable gastrointestinal tract by frequent small feedings of nutrients that are easily digested and low in residue."

This means that you will be advised to avoid any foods containing seeds, fibers, and shells, such as raw fruit, salad vegetables, nuts, or whole grains. Instead you will be advised to eat mainly such starchy and bland concoctions as cakes, spaghetti, white bread, ice cream, puddings, and dairy products. That is the conventional treatment, uniformly approved throughout the medical profession. Yet there is a very strong chance that the diet your doctor will recommend is precisely what caused your diverticulitis in the first place, and, instead of alleviating the illness, will make it worse!

Dr. Painter and two colleagues believe they have demonstrated that this low-residue diet prescribed by doctors for almost 50 years not only does not remove the symptoms of diverticular disease of the colon but is actually comprised of those foods that caused the disease to begin with.

The evidence comes in the landmark article this research team published in the *British Medical Journal.*[3] Reporting on an experiment which had been in the works for several years, the three doctors declared that of 70 patients with severe diverticular disease of the colon, 62 enjoyed marked relief of symptoms through a program of dietary change. Five others found relief through a slightly different dietary approach.

The program which helped all these people was the addition to their diet of generous amounts of natural food fiber, as found in fruit, vegetables, whole grain bread, and especially, unprocessed bran. In addition, the patients were told to reduce their intake of refined sugar in all forms.

If this sounds a little familiar, it is because some doctors, if not most, used to prescribe bran for constipation. It was safe, drugless, and it worked. But like many other answers to familiar problems, this simple and effective approach was soon replaced by more sophisticated answers which involved drugs and the direct intervention of the specialist. However, the old-time doctors who prescribed the bran for constipation probably didn't realize that it was also the best answer to much more serious intestinal ailments.

But just how effective can such a relatively simple dietary program be for people who are actually suffering? Well, here are some of the statistics published by Dr. Painter and his associates.[4] Judge for yourself:

Constipation—occurring in 28 patients before the dietary change; it was abolished in 15 and relieved in 8.

Severe colic—occurring in 12 patients before the diet; it was abolished in 7 cases and relieved in 4.

Abdominal pain—occurring in 28 patients before the diet; it was abolished in 14 cases and relieved in 11.

Tender rectum—occurring in 4 patients before the diet; it was abolished in 3 and relieved in 1.

Wind—occurring in 13 patients before the diet; it was abolished in 9 and relieved in 4 cases.

Other symptoms vanquished or markedly relieved by the high-fiber and bran diet include heartburn, nausea, bloated feeling, and incomplete emptying of the rectum. There were more benefits, Dr. Painter and his associates reported: "Before bran, 45 strained at stool, 9 did so sometimes, and only 8 defecated without effort. After bran, 51 said straining at stool was a thing of the past and only 11 had to exert themselves when emptying their bowels." Before the diet, 15 patients said they moved their bowels only every two or three days while another 13 said they were irregular. On their new dietary program, every one of the patients had a bowel movement at least once daily. Patients with the opposite problem were also helped. One poor soul who defecated 12 times a day and another who did so 6 times a day had only two movements a day on the bran diet. In other words, the dietary program relieved about nine out of ten symptoms, totally abolished irregularity, and *in every way normalized the bowel habits of most patients.*

Another recent test of bran for patients with the irritable bowel syndrome was performed by an American doctor.[5] Lt. Joseph L. Piepmeyer, in the Medical Service Corps of the United States Naval Reserve, stationed at Beaufort Naval Hospital in South Carolina, reported that 30 outpatients with the irritable bowel syndrome were selected for a test of bran. These patients, he said, had abnormal bowel habits typified by a cycle of constipation followed by the passage of hard, small stools, followed in turn by diarrhea. Many of them had varying degrees of wind and frequently suffered from abdominal bloating and cramping.

Each of the patients was instructed to take eight to ten rounded teaspoons of unprocessed bran each day, either alone or mixed with other foods. They were also warned that there is an "adjustment period" of from one to four weeks when taking bran, and they should not discontinue it if at first it made them gassy or gave them diarrhea.

It is interesting to note that Lt. Piepmeyer also took the time to explain to these patients the importance of roughage in terms of the anatomy of their bowels and to describe exactly what wheat bran is, emphasizing "the uniqueness of unprocessed bran versus other cereal products." The patients were even given recipes for using bran.

After four months on bran, 23 of the 30 outpatients reported improvement in their symptoms. Four patients withdrew from the study because they didn't like the taste of bran, so in reality, of those who actually took the bran, 90 percent improved. As was expected, their stools increased in volume, and there was also a "marked decrease in abdominal distention and cramps which was associated with some decrease in anxiety," the navy officer reported.

A diet high in roughage, or indigestible fiber, is certainly clearly indicated as a good means of preventing the formation of both "spastic colon" and diverticulitis. But what about people who already have this condition? Wouldn't a high-residue diet cause them distress?

Theoretically, it could, depending on the kind of fiber they eat. Eating a lot of seeds and nuts which have not been thoroughly chewed could conceivably cause problems.

However, when fiber is eaten in the form of bran, there are no problems. In fact, eating bran now seems to be the best thing that a person with such bowel problems can do for himself.

The reason for this is simple and is explained by Dr. T. G. Parks, a surgeon.[6] Dr. Parks told 20 patients with diverticular disease of the colon to take a small amount of bran every day, nine or ten grams, about one-third of an ounce. Previously, they had been on the "standard low-residue diet." After taking the bran, he reported, the total weight of the daily stool nearly doubled, increasing from 95 grams to 175 grams per day, a difference of 80 grams. Chemical analysis revealed that just over 80 percent of this increase consisted of water. The basic phenomenon was no surprise, because it has long been known that bran, in the gut, absorbs very large amounts of water. But Dr. Parks' work shows that *bran actually absorbs about eight times its own weight in water,* which he says, "results in the passage of more bulky, softer stools, particularly in patients previously troubled with constipation." He further says that this kind of stool is precisely what might be expected to prevent formation of high-pressure segments of the bowel from which diverticula can explode.

Drs. Painter and Burkitt have warned that diverticular disease and its complications are an increasingly serious problem in Western countries. They stress the need for preventive measures to slow the rapid climb in the number of new cases. The doctors point out that the rise in the death rate from diverticular disease was halted in England only during World War II and the years immediately following the war when there was no white bread available and white sugar was strictly rationed. Returning to the high-residue diet of the war years would probably prove a more effective cure than all the surgical treatments of today.

But Drs. Painter and Burkitt would take even

greater steps toward stamping out diverticular disease once and for all and add that, "once these causative factors have been recognized it is the duty of the profession to point the way to prevention, even if it entails issuing a warning with regard to such popular foodstuffs as white flour, both brown and white sugar, confectionery, and foods or drinks which contain unnaturally concentrated carbohydrates. Diverticular disease is a deficiency disease and, like scurvy, it should be avoidable. By retracing our dietary steps it should be possible to prevent its appearance in future generations . . . "[7]

SURGERY . . . OR BRAN?

In severe cases of diverticulitis, when the patient is in great pain and the diverticula become infected or even perforated, doctors often recommend surgery. However, many of us tend to think of surgery as a *definitive* treatment for many serious disorders, and all too frequently, at least in diverticulitis, it doesn't quite work out that way.

Doctors attending the fifth biennial congress of the International Society of Colon and Rectal Surgery in 1974 heard from Dr. Adam N. Smith, consultant surgeon at the University of Edinburgh in Scotland, the results of a long study designed to determine how beneficial bowel surgery was and if a dietary change could influence the outcome. Dr. Smith explained that if high pressures within the colon are an important factor in diverticular disease, then successful surgery will reduce these pressures, and the colon will no longer be contracting so intensely.

He decided to test the long-term usefulness of bowel surgery performed on diverticular patients by measuring colon pressures before and after their operations. He did this with two groups of patients. One group had had a portion of their large intestine removed in an operation known as a colon resection. The other group were patients who had what is known as a longitudinal myotomy, a relatively new operation in which some of the muscles which contract to create peristalsis are surgically cut.

Dr. Smith and his colleagues devised a method of measuring pressure in the colon by placing a number of surgical balloons into the bowel and recording the extent of muscular contractions. From this work, they found that patients who had undergone colon resections had no reduction at all in colon pressure following surgery. Although the sigmoid colon portion of the bowel had been removed in these patients, the problem simply moved higher up in the bowel.

In the patients who had a myotomy, muscular contractions (and therefore pressure) in the colon were considerably reduced after the operation. However, Dr. Smith and his colleagues found that this reduction only lasted for about a year. After that, it started climbing again, until after three years, it was very nearly back to what it was before surgery.

After they found that both surgical techniques for diverticular disease leave much to be desired, the Scottish surgeons set out to see if adding bran to the patients' diets would have any effect on colon pressure. Five myotomy and five resection patients were put on a daily ration of 20 grams of unprocessed bran in addition to their normal diets. (This works out to about four tablespoons of bran a day.) The patients were monitored for five years, during which time they were repeatedly subjected to tests to measure pressure in the colon. And here is what the doctors found:

Among the myotomy patients, who with surgery alone typically experienced only a one-year improvement, *the bran diet kept the pressure down during all five years of observation.* In fact, Dr. Smith said, "the colonic activity fell even lower than it did with myotomy alone and has been well maintained."

With surgery alone, patients who had undergone a colonic resection experienced only a temporary drop in pressure. But with a few tablespoons of bran every day, the drop in pressure was significant, and it remained low throughout the five years. "In light of our findings we advise giving patients bran either after a resection or a myotomy," Dr. Smith concluded.

There is no doubt that in some instances the bowel has become so damaged or infected that part of it must be surgically removed to prevent the waste products of the intestine from polluting the bloodstream with dangerous bacteria. However, there is good indication that, at least in some cases, adding bran to the diets of diverticulitis patients can actually make surgery unnecessary.

This was one of the conclusions of the earlier studies by Dr. Painter. "Twelve patients who suffered from painful diverticular disease had recurrent attacks of severe colic and *might well have come to surgery,*"Dr. Painter said, " . . . In four the colic was relieved and in seven it was abolished by the bran diet. None came to surgery despite the fact that formerly they had had attacks of severe pain. One woman of 50 had had three attacks of left renal colic . . . she was placed on a bran diet and had no further pain for two

years. Occasionally she experienced mild cramps
. . . this disappeared when she doubled her intake of
bran for a few days. *Thus even severe pain which
might have led to surgery will respond to a high-
residue diet.*"

This kind of clinical evidence points out to us that
we must *not* regard surgery as the best treatment for
bowel disease. We have seen that it is not often very effective, and in many cases it is not even necessary!
Surgery should be only a last resort—bran should
take its place as the preferred treatment for
diverticular disease.

9 | Bran, Beef, and Bowel Cancer

You may wonder why we've waited until now to discuss cancer, the most lethal of the diseases of civilization. Our intent is not to minimize the importance of the relationship between fiber and colon cancer; in fact, bran is a most valuable weapon in the war against cancer. But the subject of cancer is complex, and factors other than bran are also important considerations if we are to understand what predisposes us to bowel cancer and how we can best avoid this dread killer.

Revolutionary new research has uncovered a link between beef consumption and incidence of bowel cancer that all of us have the right to know about, for our own protection. Other research findings show that certain forms of food fiber beside bran offer us additional protection from bowel cancer.

So let's look at the problem of cancer of the colon, to find out why it has become one of the major causes of death in this country and what we can do to guard ourselves against its destructive effects.

Cancer is second only to heart disease as a cause of death in the United States. Cancer of the colon and rectum, which used to be rare in Western nations, has increased so rapidly in recent years that it now accounts for 12 to 14 percent of all cancers. In 1974, an estimated 99,000 Americans developed cancer of the colon and rectum. A year later half of them were no longer alive. "Cancer of the lower intestinal tract is the second greatest reaper in the annual death harvest from cancer," says Philip Rubin, M.D., a cancer specialist at the University of Rochester (N.Y.) Medical Center.[1] Only lung cancer kills more men and breast cancer more women. But colon cancer strikes more frequently than either lung or breast cancer; its incidence is steadily increasing and there is every indication that it will become the most lethal kind of cancer.

Yet, cancer of the colon is not so common in all parts of the world. In rural Africa, for example, colon cancer and other forms of bowel disease are practically unknown. Research has established that the illness is not the result of racial susceptibility, because black people in the United States have as much bowel cancer as whites. Instead, epidemiologists now believe that 80 percent of all cancer is probably caused by environmental factors and should be preventable. Researchers are now able to identify the most important factors in cancer causation.

Dr. Denis Burkitt, whose work was discussed in earlier chapters, has found that one important difference between Westerners who do get bowel cancer and rural Africans who don't is the length of time it takes food to pass through the digestive system (this is called intestinal transit time). Food eaten by the average Englishman takes 77 hours to pass through the gut. Tests on British vegetarians showed that they passed their food in 49 hours. But the average intestinal transit time for a rural African is a remarkably short 35 hours. And it is interesting to note that one British woman who was moving her bowels every day did not pass a marker pellet until a week after she swallowed it. So even though you may be regular on a daily basis, you may be moving food through your body very slowly.

You might wonder why transit time is important, as long as food waste is eliminated daily, but the time is indeed significant. The action of intestinal bacteria on many foods produces toxic substances that are believed to cause cancer. Processed foods may also contain carcinogenic substances in the form of certain preservatives, dyes, and artificial flavors. When wastes remain in the bowel more of these toxins are produced, and all the poisons remain in contact with the intestinal lining for a longer time and are thus more likely to do damage.

The fact that cancer of the colon (which is part of the large intestine) is widespread while cancer of the small intestine is quite rare adds further support to the idea that transit time is important in cancer. When the bowels are sluggish, decaying food is held up not in the small intestine but in the large bowel.

Constipation, one common, immediate result of delayed transit time, is also closely related to cancer of the colon. When stools are small and dry, the toxic by-products of digestion are held in a more concentrated form than if stools were large and soft. Thus, constipation may join forces with slow transit time to cause colon cancer.

In light of this combination of causes, then, the logical way to prevent colon cancer is to get rid of constipation and speed up intestinal transit time. As noted earlier, environmental factors are believed to be responsible for cancer. One of the most obvious differences between our life-style and that of rural Africans is diet, and it is to diet we must look to correct our bowel habits. We must adjust our eating habits in two ways: cut down on refined carbohydrate foods and consume more fiber.

As you know, the typical Western diet contains large amounts of fat, meats, and refined carbohydrates, and not nearly enough fruit, vegetables, and whole grains. Back in 1966, *Consumer Bulletin* reported that "the average American consumes a quarter pound per day of refined sugars, much of it in cakes, cookies, ice cream, candy, and soft drinks." And that figure is increasing all the time.

Dr. Burkitt believes that climbing rates of colon cancer parallel the climbing rates of refined carbohydrate consumption. Excess carbohydrate intake, he says, changes the bacterial content of food wastes in the intestines. Studies show that people who eat a lot of carbohydrates have an altered bacteria content which encourages the breakdown of natural bowel substances such as bile salts. In this chemical reaction, contends Dr. Burkitt, cancer-causing agents are produced.[2]

Also, since refined carbohydrates contain little roughage, they are responsible for the slow intestinal transit time which we saw earlier is related to colon cancer. As more and more refined foods have crowded supermarket shelves and household pantries, the rate of colon cancer has increased accordingly. In 1947, there were 39.3 new cases of colon cancer for every 100,000 people in the country; by 1973 the rate had jumped to 46.8 cases per 100,000 persons. Doctors are beginning to look seriously at these statistics and are concluding that the lack of dietary fiber is to blame for many of our civilized diseases.

Putting more fiber in your diet can decrease your chances of getting colon cancer in three ways. First of all, the fiber in bran and other foods helps guard your intestinal bacteria against the adverse effects of refined carbohydrates, thus inhibiting the manufacture of carcinogenic substances within your intestine. Second, fiber decreases intestinal transit time, meaning that the intestinal lining is exposed to whatever carcinogens are present for a much shorter time. And finally, the large amounts of water absorbed into your colon by the fiber dilutes the toxins and forms soft, bulky stools to put an end to constipation.

FIBER AND ENVIRONMENTAL CARCINOGENS

Of course, not all cancer-causing substances are manufactured inside our bodies. Many more come from outside sources, such as air pollutants and industrial chemicals. Some of these toxins we cannot escape, but we take many carcinogens into our bodies of our own free will! They are found in drugs and food additives—artificial colors, flavor-enhancers, preservatives. Hundreds of thousands of additives are allowed in food, and they're being developed so fast that there's no time for the FDA to properly test them all. We're putting multitudes of foreign substances into our bodies each day without knowing what effects they will ultimately have.

Fortunately, we don't have to submit to the carcinogenic effects of substances whose existence we are not even aware of. Research has now shown that fiber exerts a protective action against many kinds of toxic substances. Benjamin H. Ershoff, Ph.D., M.P.H., has found that adequate plant fiber in the diet protects laboratory animals from poisons that are fatal to animals which have been made deficient in fiber by consumption of a refined, purified diet. Dr. Ershoff concludes:

"In view of the low-fiber diets ingested by so many persons in the United States and other Western countries, serious questions arise as to whether the ingestion of drugs, chemicals, and food additives that may be without deleterious effects when ingested by persons on high-fiber diets may not constitute a hazard to health for a substantial portion of the population of these countries."[3]

The fiber-rich foods shown to be effective in countering poisons in animal experiments include wheat bran, alfalfa meal, sodium algin (a gelatinous substance extracted from seaweeds), kelp, parsley and watercress powders, powder from dried celery stalk and leaf, pectin, and various dried grasses. Also, the natural whole food stock ration for laboratory animals (as opposed to the purified fiberless diet designed for experimental purposes) contains enough fiber to be protective.

Building on this early work, Dr. Ershoff and other investigators have since shown that many harmful chemicals can be rendered harmless to research animals if fiber-rich substances are added to the diet in adequate amounts. The common food additive Tween 60 (an emulsifier, polyoxyethylene [20] sorbitan monostearate) was found toxic when given to animals at a five percent or higher proportion of a purified diet—but not when bulk-forming substances such as celluflour or agar were added to the animals' regular diet.

Similar results were obtained in the case of two other food additives: sodium cyclamate (the artificial sweetener presently banned but threatened to be restored as an approved additive in human foods) and Red No. 2 (the controversial and very widely used food-coloring chemical, amaranth, whose FDA-imposed ban was hotly challenged by the food industry).

In the case of Red No. 2, the same dose that caused death within two weeks when given to immature rats on a purified diet proved tolerable and harmless when given to immature rats along with a dietary fiber supplement—whether alfalfa meal, watercress powder, or parsley powder.

Among drugs, the diuretic chlorazanil hydrochloride, when given in high doses, caused metabolic disturbances in rats very similar to those of some humans taking this medication. But alfalfa meal added to the rats' diet largely counteracted these effects.

What is it about dietary fiber that protects against the toxic effects of these chemicals? To date, the answer remains shrouded in mystery. In early studies, it was thought that fiber simply absorbed the chemical agents and speeded their passage out of the body and that this action in itself explained the detoxification process. But this is not the whole story, as Dr. Ershoff has demonstrated in his experiments. Here's what he found:

When pure cellulose is added to a purified diet, providing the animals with adequate bulk, the toxic effects of some chemicals are reduced—but not eliminated, as they are with the addition of high-fiber foods With some chemicals (for example, the diuretic drug mentioned above) cellulose per se was found to be completely without protective effect.[4] In other words, the elusive protective factor lies hidden somewhere in natural high-fiber food—not in any known chemical fragment of the food that man can identify and duplicate in his factories.

However mysterious this natural protective factor, one thing about it is known for sure: it's been drastically reduced in the typical diet of Americans and citizens of other industrial countries.

And, if we can apply to humans what has been learned in the laboratory, our natural ability to cope with the staggering load of chemicals that affronts us today has been seriously jeopardized.

HOW BEEF HELPS TO CAUSE CANCER

Although it is not directly related to our discussion of fiber, we cannot overlook another dietary factor that has only recently been linked to cancer of the colon. A study prepared for the Pan-American Health Organization shows a wide disparity in cancer rates among Westernized countries. The bowel cancer mortality rate per 100,000 population in Bristol, England is 12.9; in La Plata, Argentina, 12.6. But the rate in Guatemala City is just 3.6; and in Cali, Columbia, only 3.3. Also, groups of people who migrate from a country like Poland—where the colon cancer rate is traditionally low—to the United States or Australia, wind up with the higher incidence rate of their adopted land after a number of years.

At first, researchers were hard-pressed to identify any one factor in the diet of Western nations that might be responsible. All these countries are relatively affluent. As a result, diets tend to be high in saturated fat, sugar, white flour, beef and other animal protein, and low in natural fiber or roughage. But as John W. Berg, M.D., and Margaret A. Howell, Ph.D., told the second National Conference on Cancer of the Colon and Rectum held in Bal Harbour, Florida, in 1973, closer investigation points directly at beef. In fact, according to Dr. Berg, "There is now substantial evidence that beef consumption is a key factor in determining bowel-cancer incidence."

The classic study which seems to clinch the case against beef was reported by Dr. Berg and four associates from the National Cancer Institute and Tohoku University School of Medicine in Japan.[5] Between 1966 and 1970, the team interviewed 179 colon cancer patients and 357 noncancer patient controls in Honolulu's three largest hospitals. All the subjects were Japanese who had been born in Japan and immigrated to Hawaii, children of immigrants, or subsequent generation Hawaiian Japanese.

The researchers found that the earliest immigrants had a higher incidence of colon cancer than later arrivals. And Hawaiian-born Japanese had the highest rates of all. But the most important factor turned out to be whether the individual had forsaken the Japanese-style diet to adopt a high-meat Western diet and for how long.

Those immigrants who had completely given up Japanese foods in favor of American-style dishes had roughly twice as much bowel cancer as those people who continued to eat at least one Japanese-style meal each day.

Most of the Japanese foods, including rice,

showed no significant statistical association with colon cancer. But among the Western foods, beef had the strongest and most dramatic correlation. In Japan, beef is seldom eaten. Pork is the predominant meat, but meats and poultry are secondary to fish and seafood. Thus, the researchers note, "Meat provides a striking example of a change in food practices between Japan and Hawaii—the rise in beef consumption—to parallel the upward displacement of bowel cancer risk among Japanese migrants."[6]

Dr. Berg and his associates pointed out that the same distinctions—although on a lesser scale—are evident among various population groups in the United States. For example, bowel cancer rates are lower in the South and among blacks. These populations eat more pork and chicken than beef. In addition, people living in cities have a higher incidence of colon cancer than those living on farms. "Beef coming to urban markets from feeding lots has a substantial fat content," the researchers report. "While the same comment would now hold true for beef supplied to rural populations through normal commercial channels, much of the beef used by farm populations in the past must have come from local slaughter of young cattle with a low fat content closely resembling that in veal."[7] Finally, the researchers point out that Seventh Day Adventists, many of whom do not eat any meat, have a death rate from intestinal cancer 20 percent below that expected.

Summing up their argument, Dr. Berg and his coworkers note, "We have found . . . no populations with a high beef intake and a low rate of bowel cancer."[8]

Meanwhile, Americans are consuming more and

more beef every year. According to statistics compiled by the American Meat Institute, the amount of beef consumed by the average American increased by 68 percent during the 20-year period ending in 1970. Per capita annual beef consumption rose from 50 pounds in 1950 to 84 pounds in 1970.[9]

BEEF AND BILE

How does increased consumption of beef trigger the development of intestinal cancer? According to British researcher Dr. M. J. Hill, high-fat, high-beef Western diets affect the lower digestive tract in two important ways. First, the level of fecal bile acids and neutral steroids is raised significantly. Two of these substances, deoxycholic acid and lithocholic acid, have been found to cause cancer in mice, says Dr. Hill, of the Bacterial Metabolism Research Laboratory of London's Central Public Health Laboratory. Second, the fatty diet increases the number of bacteria called *Clostridium paraputrificum* in the gut, which have the ability to convert certain bile acids into potent carcinogens.

Dr. Hill and his co-workers have reported that the levels of fecal bile acids and clostridia are much higher in the feces of individuals living in countries with a high-meat diet and a high evidence of colon cancer. And the levels were highest of all in newly diagnosed bowel cancer patients.[10]

In a second study, Dr. Hill suggests that if his findings are correct, "Colon cancer can be prevented by modifying the diet."[11] Vegans, who eat no meat or other sources of animal protein such as milk or eggs, have only about half the fecal bile acid concentrations of their meat-eating counterparts, he notes. While not advocating that we should all adopt such a harshly restrictive diet, Dr. Hill points out that "a mere halving of the daily fat intake to 50-60 grams/day would result in a much reduced fecal bile acid concentration while still leaving a very acceptable diet."[12]

Another very new discovery further reinforces the fact that we must cut down on our consumption of beef. A potent carcinogen present in meat itself has been identified by Raymond J. Shamberger, Ph.D., a well-known scientist in the Cleveland Clinic Foundation's biochemistry department. The substance is malonaldehyde, an extremely reactive breakdown product which begins to form in flesh almost immediately after the animal is slaughtered.

Dr. Shamberger told the annual meeting of the American Association for Cancer Research in San Diego (May 10, 1975) that he has found malonaldehyde in several types of commercially available foods. Significantly, he stated that the beef he tested had the highest levels of malonaldehyde. Samples of pork, chicken, and fish, on the other hand, had relatively low levels of the substance. And several varieties of fruit and vegetables contained very little or no malonaldehyde at all. As we might expect, leftover foods were found to contain more of this toxic breakdown product than fresh foods.

Actually, researchers have known for years that some malonaldehyde is present in beef and other meat, and even in vegetable oils and other foods under certain conditions. In fact, measurement of malonaldehyde has been used for years by the food industry as a test to determine whether or not foods are stale or rancid. But no one ever suspected that the substance could trigger cancer.

Dr. Shamberger explains malonaldehyde's effect on the human system this way: The substance, he says, "could act alone in humans or it may act in conjunction with substances such as bile acids which are known tumor promoters.

"We know that the entire human digestive system is exposed to malonaldehyde because we find it in feces," he continues. "In addition, we know that the incidence of many types of human cancer increases with age. This raises the question of whether or not human stomach, colon and other digestive tract cancers are due to a dose-response effect, i.e., an accumulation of malonaldehyde's actions in the body . . .

"If we could use just simple comparative calculations we could say that a person of average height and weight would have to consume about 15 grams of malonaldehyde to get an amount equal to the lowest dose that produced cancer in mice . . . We estimate the typical American diet contains about 1.1 grams per year or roughly 75 grams in a lifetime—comparatively far more than the mice received. It is not that simple, though, since we know that only one percent of the substance that we applied to the mice was effective— 99 percent was destroyed by the air. The amounts in the human gastrointestinal tract should not be destroyed by air and should be 100 percent effective and therefore almost 99 times as potent as the mouse doses. So, for example, by the time a person is 30 he would have consumed twice the dose we gave the mice and it may be 100 times more potent, equaling a dose of 200 times that given the mice. In a lifetime then, the dose would be five times the mouse dose, totally 500 times the potency."

SUGGESTIONS FOR PROTECTION

Fortunately, there are steps we can take to reduce the risk of malonaldehyde-induced cancer in our own lives. Dr. Shamberger and his colleagues are still working on this problem, but they offer the following preliminary suggestions:

1) Take the extra time to thaw frozen meat in the refrigerator with the wrapper intact, instead of leaving it out at room temperature. This may slow down the formation of malonaldehyde.

2) After meals, immediately wrap and cover leftover food and place it in the refrigerator.

3) Malonaldehyde is also formed during decomposition of polyunsaturated oils, and Dr. Shamberger says that people on a high-polyunsaturates diet might protect themselves by taking daily supplements of vitamins C and E. Both these nutrients are natural antioxidants which should stop the breakdown of polyunsaturated fats into malonaldehyde. Low soil concentrations of another naturally occurring antioxidant, the trace mineral selenium, are associated with higher cancer death rates in a number of American cities, Dr. Shamberger discovered in an earlier cancer research study.[13]

4) The most obvious protective measure of all is to cut down on the amount of beef and other meat you consume. You don't have to eliminate animal flesh from your diet altogether. But most Americans eat far more steak, hamburger, and roast beef sandwiches then they need to satisfy their protein or any other dietary requirement. Try a little moderation.

Remember that researchers do not yet have all the answers about cancer of the colon. While most of the evidence now points toward too much beef and too little fiber, some investigators steadfastly maintain that the responsible agent may be fat, sugar, or a combination of all these things. If you limit yourself to a *moderate* amount of beef and include some bran in your diet, you will have that much more protection.

10 | Eating Bran Can Be Grand

Now that you know why you need to use bran, the next question is how to use it. Putting bran in your diet need not be a chore. In fact, it can be a most pleasant experience, for bran can be added to many of your favorite dishes without changing taste or texture. You'll find that bran has a multitude of uses in your kitchen.

One-half cup of coarse bran can be substituted for an equal amount of flour in any recipe. You can add it to cookies, bread, muffins, cereal, or buttered toast; add it to pancakes, waffles, and french toast. Hide a teaspoonful of bran in a grilled cheese sandwich (or any other kind of sandwich).

Bran can also be added to recipes calling for bread crumbs or wheat germ. Try including bran in breading mixtures for fish, chicken, or veal cutlets, using a lower heat for the browning process. Incorporate it in casseroles and meat loaf. You can even put bran in spaghetti sauce! Just add a bit more liquid to allow for bran's absorbent quality. Bran is an all but undetectable addition to dessert toppings for apple or peach crisp, crumb cakes, and streusels. Combined with an equal amount of wheat germ, it makes a tasty garnish for a breakfast dish of fruit and yogurt. Also, if you stir-fry some with a small amount of butter until browned, it makes a nutty-flavored sprinkle for salads, cottage cheese, or other food.

Cooking with bran is easy—all it takes is a little imagination. Be creative—many of your favorite dishes can be fortified with bran. Here are some recipes to get you started on the right track.

BRAN BREAD

1 tablespoon dry yeast
1 cup lukewarm water
1 teaspoon honey
3 egg yolks
1½ tablespoons oil
3 tablespoons honey
6 tablespoons brown rice flour
6 tablespoons soy flour, sifted
6 tablespoons skim milk powder
½ teaspoon salt
¾ cup coarse bran
6 tablespoons wheat germ
½ cup raisins (optional)
3 egg whites

Oil a 9-inch-square pan. Sprinkle yeast over lukewarm water to which honey has been added. Let soak for 5 minutes. Beat egg yolks. Add oil and honey. Combine with dissolved yeast.

In a bowl, combine brown rice flour, sifted soy flour, skim milk powder, salt, bran, and wheat germ. Add raisins at this time if using them. Stir wet ingredients into dry ones. Beat egg whites until stiff but not dry. Gently fold them into batter. Turn into prepared pan and leave in a warm place for 30 minutes. Preheat oven to 375°F.

Bake bread in preheated oven for 20 to 25 minutes, or until bread tests done (inserted toothpick comes out clean).   Makes 8 servings.

BRAN MUFFINS

By all means serve warm bran muffins for breakfast. They are always welcome and so simple to prepare.

Preheat oven to 375°F.

*1 cup coarse un-
    processed bran
    flakes
1 cup whole wheat
    pastry flour
1 teaspoon salt or kelp
1 teaspoon cinnamon
2 tablespoons vegetable
    oil*

*1 cup milk
4 eggs (separated)
3 tablespoons honey or
    molasses
½ cup raisins, sun-
    flower seeds, or nuts*

Combine bran flakes and flour. Add salt or kelp and cinnamon. In another bowl, combine oil, milk, beaten egg yolks, and honey or molasses. Add to the dry ingredients. Add the raisins, seeds, or nuts or a combination of them—as you like. Beat the egg whites until stiff and fold into the batter. Bake in oiled muffin tins at 375°F. for 25 minutes. Spread with butter or cream cheese and enjoy. These muffins freeze well.

Makes 8 muffins

BRAN ENGLISH MUFFINS

Here's a tasty variation of these popular muffins.

1 tablespoon dry yeast
½ cup lukewarm water
2 teaspoons honey
1 cup milk
3 tablespoons oil
1 cup coarse bran
3 tablespoons wheat
  germ

1 teaspoon salt
1 cup unbleached flour
1 cup soy flour, sifted
1 to 1¼ cups whole
  wheat flour

Sprinkle yeast over lukewarm water to which honey has been added. Let soak for 5 minutes.

Scald milk, add oil to it and then bran, wheat germ, and salt. When this mixture has cooled to lukewarm, stir yeast mixture into it and then unbleached flour. Cover bowl and leave in a warm, draft-free spot for 1 to 1½ hours until "sponge" has doubled in bulk.

Stir "sponge" down, add sifted soy flour and 1 cup of whole wheat flour, mixing with a spoon until dough becomes too stiff. Turn out onto floured board and using as much of the remaining ¼ cup of whole wheat flour as necessary, knead dough until it is smooth and no longer sticky.

Pat or roll out dough ½-inch thick. Cut into rounds approximately 3 inches in diameter. Cover and let rest on floured surface for 45 minutes to an hour in a warm place.

Lift rounds carefully with pancake turner and bake uncovered in a lightly oiled cast-iron skillet which as been heated to medium-high heat, then turned to low. The skillet is hot enough when water hisses, if flicked onto it. Bake muffins for 10 minutes on each side until lightly browned, turning only once. Split muffins, butter and serve, or split and toast before buttering.

These muffins are worthy of a festive brunch. Try a poached egg or scrambled eggs on a bran English muffin for a real treat.

Makes 12 muffins

MUFFIN PIZZA

Delight your teenagers with these instant pizzas, supercharged with the nutrients they need for vim, vigor, and vitality.

Split bran English muffins. Top each half first with tomato sauce, then a sprinkle of oregano and garlic powder and top with mozzarella or any good-melting cheese. Place under the broiler till cheese bubbles. Serve immediately to delighted youngsters. And be sure to make some extras for yourself. They're irresistible.

BRAN COFFEE—THE CUP THAT CHEERS

Take 1 quart of bran (a ½ pound), and add enough molasses to moisten, mixing it with the hands. Spread it out in a shallow dish in a 200°F. oven. Stir it occasionally until it becomes brown (about 30 to 35 minutes). If it is inclined to be lumpy, take it out, then break up the lumps. Store in airtight containers.

If you prefer a smaller amount, use 1 cup of

bran and 4 tablespoons unsulfured molasses. The toasted granules look just like freeze-dried coffee. Add a cup of boiling water to a heaping tablespoon of these bran "coffee" globules. Add a little cream or milk, and honey if you like. Delicious—and no caffeine backlash. Then eat the moistened bran flakes which remain.

Keep these little bran-molasses granules in another bowl on your table. The children will love them just as a snack. They are crunchy and sweet and can be used as a dessert topper and instead of graham cracker crumbs for an unbaked pie crust. You could use them with seeds, raisins, and nuts as a new type of granola. Try dipping sliced bananas in these crispy crumbs.

BRAN SESAME CRACKERS

These chewy, delicious crackers make a great snack when served with your favorite dip or by themselves.

Preheat oven to 350°F.

¾ cup oatmeal
   ("ground" in
   blender a bit so that
   it resembles coarse
   oat flour)
½ cup coarse bran
1 cup whole wheat
   flour

½ teaspoon salt
6 tablespoons oil
1 tablespoon honey
½ cup water
¼ cup sesame seeds

Combine dry ingredients. Combine oil, honey, and water and stir into dry mixture. Grease a cookie sheet generously. Pat dough out on the cookie sheet and roll it with a rolling pin until it is as thin as possible (⅛ inch). Sprinkle sesame seeds over the surface and roll them into the dough with the rolling pin. Score the dough with a knife in squares or diamonds in whatever size you wish. Bake 10 to 12 minutes in preheated 350°F. oven. Loosen crackers with a spatula as soon as they are removed from the oven. Cool and store in an airtight container.

Makes 4 dozen crackers, approximately 2-inch squares

BRAN COOKIES

Children and grown-ups alike will go for these flavorful cookies.

Preheat oven to 350°F.

1½ cups whole wheat
    flour
3 cups coarse bran
½ teaspoon salt
1 teaspoon ginger
1 teaspoon cinnamon
½ teaspoon cloves
2 eggs
½ cup oil

½ cup honey
½ cup milk
½ raisins (other
    chopped dried
    fruit may be
    substituted)
½ cup chopped nuts
    (optional)

Combine dry ingredients. Beat eggs, then add oil, honey, and milk to them and blend together. Stir the wet ingredients into the dry, add raisins and nuts if using them. Drop by teaspoonfuls, 2 inches apart on a greased cookie sheet. Bake in a preheated 350°F. oven for 8 to 10 minutes. Watch cookies carefully as these tend to brown quickly on the bottom.

Makes 4 dozen cookies

CARROT CAROB BRAN CAKE

A delicious, not-too-sweet cake which goes well with coffee and can be eaten just as it is, or it can be topped with cream cheese, or cottage cheese mixed with yogurt, and chopped nuts.

Preheat oven to 350°F.

½ cup raisins
⅔ cup hot water
1 cup finely grated carrots
2 egg yolks
3 tablespoons carob, sifted
¼ cup soy flour, sifted

¾ cup whole wheat flour
¾ teaspoon cinnamon
¼ teaspoon salt
grated rind of 1 lemon
½ cup coarse bran
2 egg whites

Combine raisins and hot water in a bowl. Add grated carrot, egg yolks, sifted carob, sifted soy flour, whole wheat flour, cinnamon, salt, and lemon rind. Finally add the bran, stirring to blend together. Beat egg whites stiff and fold into mixture. Turn into oiled pie pan (9 inch), or if using a bread pan (large size), line it first with oiled brown paper. Bake in preheated 350°F. oven for 35 to 40 minutes. Remove from oven. If bread pan was used, removed cake from pan after about 10 minutes, and strip off paper. Cake can remain in pie plate until serving time.

Makes 6 to 8 servings

BANANA-NUT BREAD

Preheat oven to 375°F.

2½ cups soft, ripe
   bananas
1 egg
¼ cup oil
¼ to ⅓ cup honey
¾ cup bran
4 tablespoons water
½ teaspoon salt
2 teaspoons baking
   powder

½ teaspoon baking
   soda
3 cups unbleached
   flour
1 teaspoon vanilla ex-
   tract
½ cup chopped nuts

Peel and mash bananas and set aside. Beat egg in a large bowl until light and foamy. Mix oil and honey with the beaten egg, then stir in bran, water, and bananas; mix well. Sift the remaining dry ingredients, then slowly add to the banana mixture, stirring constantly. Add vanilla extract and nuts, and mix until smooth. Bake in a well-oiled loaf pan at 375°F. for 1 hour.

Makes 1 loaf

PEANUT BUTTER SESAME BALLS

Great for parties . . . or just for snacking.

Preheat oven to 200°F.

¾ cup peanut butter
½ cup honey
1 teaspoon pure vanilla
    extract
¾ cup skim milk
    powder
⅓ cup bran
⅔ cup oatmeal

¼ cup toasted sesame
    seeds*
2 tablespoons boiling
    water
chopped nuts or
    toasted sesame seeds
    for coating balls

In a medium-sized bowl, combine peanut butter, honey, and vanilla extract; blend thoroughly. Mix skim milk powder, bran, and oatmeal together. Gradually add to the peanut butter-honey mixture, blending thoroughly, using hands if necessary to mix as dough begins to stiffen. Blend in the toasted sesame seeds. Add boiling water to mixture, blending well.

Shape in 1-inch balls. Roll in finely chopped nuts or toasted sesame seeds. For variety, roll half the mixture in chopped nuts and the other half in toasted sesame seeds.

*Toast sesame seeds in a preheated 200°F. oven for about 20 minutes or until lightly browned.

Makes approximately 3 dozen balls

APPLE CRISP

An all-time favorite dessert—made better!

Preheat oven to 375°F.

4 to 6 baking apples,
peeled and cored
⅔ cup brown sugar,
packed
¼ cup whole wheat
flour

¼ cup bran
⅓ cup rolled oats
¾ teaspoon cinnamon
¾ teaspoon nutmeg
⅓ cup soft butter

Slice apples into an oiled, 8-inch-square baking dish. Combine remaining ingredients and sprinkle over apples. Bake at 375°F. for 30 to 35 minutes, or until top is golden brown.

Makes 6 servings

SNACKIN' BANANAS

Try these for a midmorning pickup or a nutritious bedtime snack.

3 teaspoons bran
3 teaspoons wheat
germ

6 peeled, ripe bananas
peanut butter

Mix bran and wheat germ together and set aside. Cut bananas into 3-inch pieces so they're easier to work with. Split each piece in half, lengthwise, and spread one half with peanut butter. Press halves together and roll in the bran-wheat germ mixture.

Any number of bananas can be made; just allow approximately ½ teaspoon of bran and ½ teaspoon of wheat germ for each banana.

HOMEMADE IS THE BEST BRAND OF CEREAL

What's your favorite kind of cereal? Do you most enjoy the Swiss Muesli cereals, replete with dried fruit and roasted nuts? Do you prefer the sweet and crunchy granolas now offered at most supermarkets? Or do you think a hot, cooked cereal the most satisfying way to start a cold morning? Without much effort, you can create a variety of cereals exactly to your own tastes and surpassing the supermarket's in quality, flavor, and nutrition. If you make your own cereals, you can be sure they contain lots of fiber without the empty calories of refined sugar.

Most health food stores offer a variety of natural ingredients for concocting your own cereals. Among the grains you might choose from are rolled oats and wheat germ, or rye, wheat, millet, and rice in flakes and flours, as well as cornmeal and, of course, rolled bran. Your own garden might offer sunflower, squash, and pumpkin seeds to supplement the health food store's sesame seeds and their cashews, pecans, walnuts, almonds, hazelnuts, and peanuts. You could add raisins, chopped dates and prunes, snipped figs and apricots, or dried peaches, apples, and pears (from your own garden perhaps?). You may find that your prefer no other sweetening than that naturally present in the fruit and grains, or you could try adding honey, molasses, maple syrup, or date sugar.

SWISS MUESLI

For an untoasted Swiss-type cereal you start with 2 parts rolled or oat flakes. Now add 1 part wheat germ, 1 part of another flaked or rolled grain, and 1 part coarse bran. Hazelnuts and almonds characterize the traditional cereal, but you can choose any combination of nuts or seeds which appeals to you and add 1 to 2 parts. If desired, you could first toast them in a 300°F. oven, turning frequently to prevent scorching until very lightly browned. You can add 1 part (or more) raisins and 1 part of another dried fruit chopped into bite-sized pieces, or you can add fresh fruit at the table. Before storing you could sweeten the mixture with date sugar, or plan on serving it with honey or maple syrup, or simply rely on the sweetness of the fruit. Store your cereal in a covered container in the refrigerator. By adding instant milk powder (about ⅓ cup for each cup of cereal), you'll have a lightweight but satisfying campsite breakfast that requires only the addition of water. At home, serve it with milk, yogurt, buttermilk, or fruit juice.

CRUNCHY GRANOLA

For a crunchy granola-type cereal, start with 3 parts rolled oats, 1 part of another flaked grain or mixture of grains, 1 part bran, 1 part nuts, 1 part seeds, and 1 part unsweetened dry coconut shreds. You could boost its nutritional value with soy grits (about ½ part) or a little brewer's yeast or powdered milk. Combine ¼ part oil, ½ part water, and a little vanilla if you desire. Add to dry ingredients, stirring until grains and nuts are well coated. Pour the mixture into a large, shallow baking pan which has been lightly oiled and toast in a low oven (250°F.) for 1 to 1½ hours, stirring every 10 to 15 minutes or until mixture is dry and lightly browned and crisp. Remove the cereal from the oven, and allow it to cool. Add 1 to 2 parts raisins or other dried fruit. Store in a plastic bag or jar in the refrigerator.

CREAM OF WHEAT, RYE, OR RICE

Everyone is familiar with oatmeal as a rib-sticking, cold-weather, warm-up breakfast. Perhaps you've also had other cooked cereals, but have you ever tried making your own cream of wheat, rye, or rice to fight the shivers on frosty mornings? It's a simple process of "popping" the whole grains in a dry frying pan over medium heat and then grinding them coarse or fine, according to how crunchy or creamy your family prefers its hot cereals.

There's no need to cover the frying pan as you do when popping corn; just shake gently to prevent scorching until all the grains have browned and smell nutty. Grind the popped grains in a blender or a home grain mill. After grinding you can toast the grains lightly again if you wish. Store cooled ground grains in a tightly covered jar in the refrigerator.

To prepare 4 servings, bring 5 cups of milk and 1 teaspoon of salt to a boil, then stir in 1 cup of the ground grains and a ¼ cup of bran. Lower the heat, cover the pan, and allow it to simmer 5 to 10 minutes, or until the cereal is as thick as you wish. You could also add brewer's yeast, wheat germ, sesame or sunflower seeds, ground or chopped nuts, milk, butter, honey, molasses or maple syrup, and dried or fresh fruit. More cereal recipes follow.

HOT RAISIN BRAN

Here's a cold-weather version of a summertime favorite.

3 cups water
½ teaspoon salt
⅓ cup wheat germ
⅔ cup bran

¼ cup nonfat dry milk
*   powder*
2 tablespoons raisins

Bring water to a boil in a heavy-bottomed saucepan. Stir in remaining ingredients and cook gently, uncovered, for 10 minutes, stirring occasionally. Serve with additional milk, plus honey or molasses to taste.

Makes 4 servings

BREAD CEREAL

Whole wheat in the form of whole wheat bread is the basis of this cereal. (It's a good way to use stale bread.)

3 cups diced whole
*   grain bread (about 8*
*   slices or ½ lb.)*
4 cups milk, whole or
*   skim*

¼ cup wheat germ
¼ cup bran
½ teaspoon salt

In a heavy-bottomed saucepan, combine all ingredients and bring to boil over moderate heat, stirring constantly. Reduce heat and cook gently uncovered, mashing bread with a fork, 3 to 5 minutes or until thickened. Serve with additional milk if desired, and raisins, chopped nuts, or other cereal garnish.

Makes 4 large servings

GAZPACHO SOUP

2 garlic cloves, crushed
1 teaspoon salt
½ teaspoon powdered
   pepper
pulp of 2 tomatoes
4 tablespoons olive oil
2 tablespoons fresh
   breadcrumbs
2 tablespoons bran
1 large onion, thinly
   sliced

1 sweet pepper, red or
   green (remove seeds
   and pulp and dice)
1 cucumber (peel,
   remove seeds, and
   dice)
3 cups cold water
1 tablespoon vinegar
   (optional)

Mix the garlic, salt, pepper, and the tomato
pulp thoroughly in a blender at low speed. Add
the olive oil drop by drop through the hole in the
blender cap until an emulsion forms. Using the
lowest speed, blend in breadcrumbs, bran, onion,
and the rest of the ingredients. Serve very cold.

Makes 4 servings

CRUSTY OVEN-BAKED FISH

Preheat oven to 400°F.

2 lbs. haddock or
   flounder fillets
½ cup wheat germ
½ cup peanut flour
   (raw peanuts
   ground in blender or
   nut grinder)
¼ cup sesame seeds
½ cup bran flakes
1 teaspoon salt

½ teaspoon black pep-
   per
½ teaspoon oregano
½ teaspoon marjoram
½ teaspoon paprika
½ teaspoon garlic
   powder
1 egg, beaten
½ cup oil
½ cup lemon juice

Rinse fish. Cut into portions and leave to
drain. Combine all dry ingredients to make

crumb mixture and set aside. Combine egg, oil, and lemon juice in a blender or use an eggbeater to obtain an emulsion. Dip portions of fish into egg dip and then into crumb mixture. Lay on shallow baking pan which has been lightly oiled. Bake in preheated 400°F. oven approximately 20 minutes, until tender.

Makes 6 to 8 servings

ITALIAN MEATBALLS WITH SAUCE

⅓ cup minced onion
1 garlic clove, minced
   (optional)
1 tablespoon olive oil
¼ cup potato flour or
   brown rice flour
1 ½ tablespoons corn-
   starch
½ cup water
2 eggs, slightly beaten
1 ½ lbs. beef (ground
   round) or ½ lb.
   ground veal may be
   used with 1 lb.
   ground round

¼ cup raw wheat germ
2 tablespoons bran
2 tablespoons fresh
   parsley, chopped
   fine
1 teaspoon salt
¼ teaspoon ground
   pepper
⅓ cup Romano or
   Parmesan cheese
   (grated)

Sauté minced onion and garlic in oil until golden but not brown. In a small mixing bowl, combine flour, cornstarch, and water, making a smooth paste. Add beaten eggs and mix thoroughly. In a large mixing bowl, combine meat and sautéed onion and garlic. Next add beaten eggs and starch mixture, then wheat germ, bran, parsley, salt, pepper, and grated cheese. Mix ingredients thoroughly. Form meat mixture into balls about 2 inches in diameter. Brown meatballs under broiler, turning them as they brown. Remove and set aside.

Makes 4 to 6 servings or approximately 24 meatballs

SAUCE

1 onion, chopped (approximately ⅔ cup)
1 garlic clove, minced
2 tablespoons olive oil
3 cups fresh or canned tomatoes
2 cups tomato puree
1 teaspoon crushed oregano
¼ teaspoon crushed basil
1½ teaspoons salt
2 teaspoons honey

In a 4-quart container, sauté onion and garlic in olive oil until golden but not brown. Stir in tomatoes, tomato puree, oregano, basil, salt, and honey. Simmer sauce, uncovered, for 30 minutes. Add browned meatballs and continue to simmer 45 minutes longer; adjust seasonings. Note: This dish may be served with spaetzle, polenta, or brown rice.

Makes approximately 4 cups

VEGETABLE-BEEF LOAF

Preheat oven to 350°F.

1 onion, chopped (⅓ cup)
1 garlic clove, minced
⅓ cup green pepper, chopped
⅓ cup celery, chopped
½ cup shredded carrot
1 tablespoon oil
3 tablespoons soy grits
⅔ cup tomato juice
1 lb. ground beef (chuck or round)
⅔ lb. ground beef heart (if heart is not available, substitute ½ lb. ground beef)

1 egg, beaten
2 tablespoons wheat germ
2 tablespoons bran
2 tablespoons nutritional yeast
2 tablespoons soy flour (sifted)
3 tablespoons chopped parsley
2 tablespoons catsup
⅓ teaspoon salt
⅓ teaspoon pepper
⅓ teaspoon thyme
⅓ teaspoon basil

Sauté onion, garlic, green pepper, celery, and carrot in oil. Soak soy grits in tomato juice for about 15 minutes. Combine meat, egg, wheat germ, bran, nutritional yeast, soy flour, parsley, catsup, and seasonings. Add sautéed vegetable mixture and the soy grits and tomato mixture. Mix well.

Oil 9 x 5 x 3-inch loaf pan, bottom and sides, and press meat mixture into pan. Bake at 350°F. for 1 hour or until meat is cooked at center. Turn out of loaf pan, slice, and serve.

Makes 6 to 8 servings

MOLDED MEAT LOAF WITH OATMEAL

Preheat oven to 350°F.

2 lbs. lean ground beef
(chuck or round)
⅓ cup wheat germ
1 cup oatmeal
¼ cup bran
2 tablespoons freshly
chopped parsley
½ teaspoon freshly
ground pepper

1 teaspoon salt
½ cup chopped onion
2 tablespoons oil
2 eggs
¼ cup skim milk
powder
½ cup water
½ cup tomato juice

In a large mixing bowl, combine ground beef, wheat germ, oatmeal, bran, chopped parsley, pepper, and salt; set aside. Sauté onion in oil until tender but not brown; add to meat. Beat eggs lightly. Combine skim milk powder and water with a wire whisk, and add to eggs. Blend together and add to meat mixture; then add tomato juice. Mix thoroughly.

Oil a 9 x 5 x 3-inch loaf pan. Turn meat mixture into pan, packing down well. Allow to rest 10 to 15 minutes in refrigerator. Run spatula around edge of meat loaf to loosen. Carefully turn out into a lightly oiled shallow baking pan, keeping original shape as much as possible. Brush surface with oil. Place meat loaf on middle rack of a preheated 350°F. oven and bake for 1¼ hours. Remove from oven when nicely browned and allow to rest 10 minutes before serving.

Makes 6 to 8 servings

SUNBURGERS

A truly delicious meatless entree.

Preheat oven to 350°F.

½ cup grated raw car-
  rots
½ cup celery, chopped
  fine
2 tablespoons chopped
  onion
1 tablespoon chopped
  parsley
1 tablespoon chopped
  green pepper

1 egg, beaten
1 tablespoon oil
¼ cup tomato juice
¾ cup ground sun-
  flower seeds
¼ cup bran
2 tablespoons wheat
  germ
½ teaspoon salt
⅛ teaspoon basil

Combine ingredients and shape into patties.
Arrange in an oiled, shallow baking dish. Bake in
a moderate oven (350°F.) until brown on top;
turn patties and bake until brown. (Allow about
15 minutes of baking for each side.)

Makes approximately 4 servings

STUFFED EGGS

6 eggs
2 tablespoons mayon-
  naise
½ teaspoon mustard
½ teaspoon cider (or
  wine) vinegar
½ teaspoon salt
dash of pepper

4 green onions
2 tablespoons green
  pepper
1 teaspoon chopped
  chives
2 tablespoons sun-
  flower seeds
1 tablespoon bran

Hard-cook eggs. Crack and drop immediately into cold water. Shell and cut in half

lengthwise. Separate yolks from whites. Reserve egg whites. Put egg yolks and rest of ingredients in blender. When completely combined and smooth, refill egg whites with the mixture.

Makes 12 egg halves

BAKED TOMATOES

Preheat oven to 350°F.

4 large tomatoes
½ cup dark
  breadcrumbs
¼ cup bran
3 tablespoons chopped
  young onion
3 garlic cloves, crushed
4 tablespoons chopped
  fresh basil

4 parsley sprigs
½ teaspoon dried
  thyme
salt and pepper to taste
1 tablespoon tomato
  paste (optional)
grated cheese
olive oil

Cut a circle out of the stem end of each tomato, carefully cut out the pulp, and drain the shells. Combine the pulp with the breadcrumbs, bran, onions, garlic, and herbs. Add salt and pepper to taste. If these ingredients don't make a good thick paste, add tomato paste. Fill the shells, then top with grated cheese. Oil a casserole and arrange the tomatoes in it. Bake at 350°F. for 30 minutes or until tops are brown and cheese is melted. Serve immediately.

Makes 4 servings

STUFFED EGGPLANT

Preheat oven to 350°F.

2 eggplants, split in
  half lengthwise
1 medium-sized onion,
  chopped
½ garlic clove, minced
2 tablespoons oil
½ lb. cooked beef, cut
  in small cubes
2 cups tomatoes (fresh
  or canned)

salt to taste
3 tablespoons bran
½ teaspoon basil
2 tablespoons wheat
  germ
3 tablespoons
  Parmesan cheese

Scoop pulp from eggplant halves, leaving ½-inch shell. Dice pulp. Sauté onion, garlic, and eggplant pulp in oil. Add cubed, cooked meat, tomatoes, salt (to taste), bran, and basil. Fill eggplant shells with mixture; top with wheat germ combined with cheese.

Put water ½-inch deep in bottom of baking pan. Add filled eggplant halves, cover with foil and bake at 350°F. for 30 minutes. Then uncover and continue baking until shell is tender enough to eat (about 20 minutes).

Makes 6 to 8 servings

TOMATO SAUCE

2 tablespoons olive oil
½ onion, chopped
2 garlic cloves, crushed
1 tablespoon chopped
  green pepper
28-ounce can Italian
  paste tomatoes
½ lb. ground meat

1 tablespoon bran
1 tablespoon parsley
1 teaspoon basil or
  oregano
1 small bay leaf
salt and pepper as
  desired
water (or red wine)

Heat the oil in a large frying pan and sauté the onion and garlic. Stir in the pepper and tomato and simmer 2 minutes. Transfer all to a blender and blend at a fairly high speed for 1 minute. In the meantime, brown the ground meat in the empty frying pan until no red shows. Then pour the blended sauce over the meat, add the bran and herbs, and simmer for 30 minutes or longer. (The longer you simmer it, the better it tastes.) Add water or red wine if it boils down. Serve with spaghetti or other pasta.

Appendixes

APPENDIX A: FIBER AND CARBOHYDRATE CONTENT OF COMMON FOODS

In deciding which foods to include in your diet to supply you with fiber, you must consider not only the actual fiber content but also the proportion of fiber to total carbohydrates (remember that fiber is a part of carbohydrates—the part your body cannot digest and burn for energy). Some foods, such as pretzels, contain appreciable amounts of fiber, but the huge amounts of carbohydrates and calories they contain make them an unwise choice as a source of fiber. The ideal roughage foods contain a large proportion of fiber to total carbohydrates (see wheat bran); the ones to avoid contain little or no fiber and large quantities of carbohydrates (see sugar).

This chart is an alphabetical listing of common foods with their content of fiber, total carbohydrates, and calories (a measure of the amount of energy the carbohydrates provide for the human body). Take note that when a good proportion of fiber to total carbohydrates exists, a seemingly large amount of calories won't prove as fattening; the fiber prevents your body from absorbing all the calories. Also bear in mind that while cooking vegetables may lower their calorie value, many vitamins are also lost in the process. When rating foods as fiber sources, compare them with crude wheat bran as the best source of fiber and granulated white sugar as the worst.

The information for this chart was taken from *Composition of Foods*, USDA Agriculture Handbook No. 8. Figures are in terms of 100-gram portions (approximately three and one-half ounces) of food.

Food	Calories	Carbohydrate Total	Fiber
Apples, unpared	60	14.8	1.0
Applesauce, sweetened	75.7	23.8	.5
Apricots			
raw	51	12.8	.6
canned in heavy syrup	86	22.0	.4
Blackberries			
canned in water	40	9.0	2.8
juice	37	7.8	trace
Blueberries			
raw	62	15.3	1.5
canned in heavy syrup	101	26.0	
Boysenberries			
canned in water	36	9.1	1.9
Bread			
pumpernickel	246	53.1	1.1
white, enriched	270	50.5	.2
whole wheat	243	47.7	1.6
Chocolate cake w/choc. icing	369	55.8	.3
Candies			
gumdrops	347	87.4	0
hard candy	386	97.2	0
milk chocolate	520	56.9	.4
Carrots			
raw	42	9.7	1.0
boiled, drained	31	7.1	1.0

Food	Calories	Carbohydrate Total	Fiber
Cauliflower			
raw	27	5.2	1.0
boiled, drained	22	4.1	1.0
Celery			
raw	17	3.9	.6
boiled, drained	14	3.1	.6
Cookies			
chocolate chip	516	60.1	.4
sugar	444	68.0	.1
Corn on cob, cooked	91	21.0	.7
Cornmeal			
degermed, enriched	364	78.4	.6
wholeground, unbolted	355	73.7	1.6
Corn pone (whole meal)	204	36.2	.8
Crackers			
cheese	479	60.4	.2
graham, plain	384	73.3	1.1
graham, sugar/honey	411	76.4	.8
whole wheat	403	68.2	2.4
Cranberries			
raw	46	10.8	1.4
canned, sauce	146	37.5	.2
Cucumbers			
raw, pared	14	3.2	.3
Doughnuts			
yeast-leavened	414	37.7	.2
Eggplant			
raw	25	5.6	.9
boiled, drained	19	4.1	.9
Figs			
raw	80	20.3	1.2
canned in heavy syrup	84	21.8	.7
Filberts	634	16.7	3.0
Ice cream			
regular, approx. 10% fat	193	20.8	0
rich, approx. 16% fat	222	18.0	0
Macaroni			
enriched, cooked	148	20.1	.1
Milk			
whole (w/national average of 3.7% fat)	66	4.9	0

Food	Calories	Carbohydrate Total	Fiber
Muffins			
bran (enriched flour)	261	43.1	1.8
plain (enriched flour)	294	42.3	.1
Pancakes			
buckwheat	200	23.8	.4
enriched flour	231	34.1	.1
Peaches			
raw	38	9.7	.6
canned in heavy syrup	78	20.1	.4
dried	262	68.3	3.1
Peanut butter			
fat & salt added	581	17.2	1.9
Pears			
raw	61	15.3	1.4
canned in heavy syrup	76	19.6	.6
dried	268	67.3	6.2
Peas (green)			
boiled, drained	71	12.1	2.0
split, cooked	115	20.8	.4
Pepper (green)			
raw	22	4.8	1.4
boiled, drained	18	3.8	1.4
Pies			
apple	256	38.1	.4
blackberry	243	34.4	1.9
custard	218	23.4	trace
Popcorn			
plain	386	76.7	2.2
sugar-coated	383	85.4	1.1
Potatoes			
baked in skin	93	21.1	.6
instant granules, prepared	96	14.4	.2
Potato chips	568	50.1	1.6
Pretzels	390	75.9	.3
Prunes			
dried	255	67.4	1.6
juice	77	19.0	.3
Puddings			
homemade chocolate	148	25.7	.2
homemade vanilla	111	15.9	trace

Food	Calories	Carbohydrate Total	Fiber
instant chocolate	125	24.1	.1
Raisins	289	77.4	.9
Raspberries			
raw black	73	15.7	5.1
raw red	57	13.6	3.0
Rice (cooked)			
brown	119	25.5	.3
enriched white	109	24.2	.1
instant white	109	24.2	.1
Rice cereal (cooked)	50	11.2	2.4
Rice polish	265	57.7	2.4
Rice pudding (w/raisins)	146	26.7	.1
Rolls			
plain, enriched	298	53.0	.2
sweet	316	49.3	.2
whole wheat	257	52.3	1.6
Rye flour			
light	357	77.9	.4
medium	350	74.8	1.0
dark	327	68.1	2.4
Rye wafers	344	76.3	2.2
Sauerkraut	18	4.0	.7
Sesame seeds, whole	563	21.6	6.3
Soybeans			
boiled, drained	118	10.1	1.4
Soybean curd (tofu)	72	2.4	.1
Soybean flour			
low fat	356	36.6	2.5
high fat	380	33.3	2.2
Spaghetti			
enriched, cooked	148	20.1	.1
Spinach			
raw	26	4.3	.6
boiled, drained	23	3.6	.6
canned	19	3.0	.7
frozen, boiled, drained	24	3.9	.8
Squash			
acorn			
baked	55	14.0	1.8
boiled, mashed	34	8.4	1.4

Food	Calories	Carbohydrate Total	Fiber
butternut			
baked	68	17.5	1.8
boiled, mashed	41	10.4	1.4
zucchini, boiled & drained	12	2.5	.6
Sugar (beet and cane)			
brown	373	96.4	0
granulated white	385	99.5	0
powdered	385	99.5	0
Sweet potatoes			
baked in skin	141	32.5	.9
candied	168	34.2	.6
Table syrup			
mostly corn, light or dark	290	75.0	0
Tapioca pudding	134	17.1	0
Tomatoes			
raw	22	4.7	.5
boiled, drained	26	5.5	.6
canned	21	4.3	.4
catsup	106	25.4	.5
juice	19	4.3	.2
Turnips			
boiled, drained	23	4.9	.9
Walnuts			
black	628	14.8	1.7
English	651	15.8	2.1
Watermelon	26	6.4	.3
Wheat bran			
crude, commercially milled	213	61.9	9.1
with sugar & defatted germ	238	78.8	6.5
40% flakes	303	80.6	3.6
Wheat flour			
enriched white	364	76.1	.3
white pastry	364	79.4	.2
whole grain	333	71.0	2.3

APPENDIX B: FIBER DEPLETION IN REFINED FOODS

As we know, a whole food contains more fiber than the same food in a refined form, and the com-

parative listing below of the actual amounts of fiber in
a group of whole and processed foods dramatically
illustrates just how much fiber is really lost.

These figures are also from *Composition of Foods*
and were calculated in terms of 100-gram portions of
food.

Whole food	grams fiber	Refined food	grams fiber
Apples	1.0	applesauce	.5
Bread whole wheat	1.6	white, enriched	.2
Cornmeal whole	1.6	degermed	.6
Cranberries raw	1.4	cranberry sauce	.2
Graham crackers plain	1.1	with sugar and honey	.8
Muffins bran	1.8	plain (enriched flour).	.1
Pears raw	1.4	canned in heavy syrup	.6
Popcorn plain	2.2	sugar-coated	1.1
Potatoes whole, baked	.6	instant	.2
Prunes dried	1.6	juice	trace
Rolls whole wheat	1.6	plain (enriched flour)	.2
Rye flour dark	2.4	light	.4
Wheat bran crude	9.1	with sugar & defatted germ	6.5
Wheat flour whole	2.3	enriched white	.3

APPENDIX C: FIBER AND REFINED SUGAR CONTENT OF CEREALS

Since we now know that whole grains and bran contain fiber, it seems only natural to turn to grain products such as breakfast cereals to supply us with fiber. You may think that since these are *breakfast* cereals, vitamin-fortified and containing appreciable amounts of fiber, they must be good for you. But these refined products are loaded with sugar in huge amounts that practically negate the benefits of the fiber.

Many of these cereals contain more sugar than candy! Scientific analysis of cereal content has shown that 40 percent of our major commercial cereal products are at least one-third sugar.[1] The average amount of sugar in candies is 37.1 percent—lower than the amount in many breakfast cereals. Starting your day with these sugar-coated, fruit-flavored cereals is like eating candy for breakfast. In terms of bowel health, you'd be much better off with less glamorous foods like good old-fashioned oatmeal (not the instant kind) or granola you make yourself with rolled oats, nuts, raisins, and no sugar.

The chart shows approximate grams of fiber per 100 grams of cereal and the percentage of the product which is refined sugar. Amounts of fiber were taken from the *Medical Letter*, November 23, 1973. Sugar percentages are from the *Journal of Dentistry for Children*, September-October 1974.

Cereal	grams fiber	Name of product	% sugar
Corn	.2-.4	Post Toasties	4.1
		Corn Total	4.4

Cereal	grams fiber	Name of product	% sugar
	.2-.4	Kellogg's Corn Flakes	7.8
		Sugar Frosted Flakes	15.6
		Sugar Pops	37.8
		Cocoa Puffs	43.0
		Trix	46.6
Rice	.2-.4	Puffed Rice	2.4
		Rice Krispies	10.0
		Cocoa Krispies	45.9
Mixed	.3-.5	Product 19	4.1
		Special K	4.4
		Kellogg's Concentrate	9.9
		Froot Loops	42.4
		Kaboom	43.8
		Frankenberry	44.0
		Count Chocula	44.2
		Apple Jacks	55.0
Oats	.6-1.2	Cheerios	2.2
		Fortified Oat Flakes	22.2
		Lucky Charms	50.4
Wheat & Barley	1.8	Grape-Nuts Flakes	3.3
		Grape Nuts	6.6
Wheat	1.1-2.3	Shredded Wheat	1.0
		Puffed Wheat	3.5
		Wheaties	4.7
		Total	8.1
		Buckwheats	13.6
		Sugar Smacks	61.3
Bran	2.7-3.8	Kellogg's Raisin Bran	10.6
		Post's 40% Bran Flakes	15.8
		Kellogg's 40% Bran Flakes	16.2
		Kellogg's All-bran	20.0
		Bran Buds	30.2

Notes

Notes, Chapter 1

1. (p. 2) William B. Seaman, Address to meeting of the Radiological Society of North America, reported in *Radiology*, August 1971.

Notes, Chapter 3

1. (p. 28) Information on types and brands of laxatives appeared in "Laxatives and Dietary Fiber," *Medical Letter* 15 (November 23, 1973): 98–100.
2. (p. 32) See note 1 above.
3. (p. 36) Thomas L. Cleave, Letter to the Editor, *British Medical Journal* 2 (May 13, 1972): 408–409.
4. (p. 39) Neil S. Painter, Anthony Z. Almeida, and Kenneth W. Colebourne, "Unprocessed Bran in Treatment of Diverticular Disease of the Colon," *British Medical Journal* 2 (April 15, 1972): 137–140.

Notes, Chapter 6

1. (p. 56) Kenneth W. Heaton, "Are We Getting Too Much Out of Food?" (Lecture to the West of England and South Wales Branch of the British Dietetic Association,

December 7, 1972). Reprinted from *Nutrition, London* 27, no. 3 (1973): 170–183. Printed in Great Britain.

2. (p. 59) Stephen B. Hulley et al, "Lipid and Lipoprotein Responses of Hypertriglyceridemic Outpatients to a Low-Carbohydrate Modification of the A.H.A. Fat-Controlled Diet," *Lancet* 2 (September 16, 1972): 551–555.

3. (p. 62) Heaton, "Food Fiber As An Obstacle to Energy Intake," *Lancet* 2 (December 22, 1971): 1418–1421.

4. (p. 63) Thomas L. Cleave, "The Neglect of Natural Principles in Current Medical Practice," *Journal of the Royal Navy Medical Service* 42 (Spring 1956): 55–83.

5. (p. 64) Hugh C. Trowell, "Dietary-fiber Hypothesis of the Etiology of Diabetes Mellitus," *Diabetes* 24 (August 1975): 762–765.

6. (p. 65) "Roughage In The Diet," *Medical World News* 15 (September 6, 1974): 35–42.

7. (p. 66) See note 6 above.

Notes, Chapter 7

1. (p. 69) Denis P. Burkitt and Peter A. James, "Low-Residue Diets and Hiatus Hernia," *Lancet* 2 (July 21, 1973): 128–130.

2. (p. 70) Burkitt, A.R.P. Walker, and Neil S. Painter, "Dietary Fiber and Disease," *Journal of the American Medical Association* 229 (August 19, 1974): 1068–1074.

Notes, Chapter 8

1. (p. 75) Neil S. Painter and Denis P. Burkitt, "Diverticular Disease of the Colon: A Deficiency Disease of Western Civilization," *British Medical Journal* 2 (May 22, 1971): 450–454.

2. (p. 76) See note 1 above.

3. (p. 77) Painter, Anthony Z. Almeida, and Kenneth W. Colebourne, "Unprocessed Bran in Treatment of Diverticular Disease of the Colon," *British Medical Journal* 2 (April 15, 1972): 137–140.

4. (p. 78) See note 3 above.

5. (p. 79) Joseph L. Piepmeyer, Letter to the Editor, *American Journal of Clinical Nutrition* 27 (February 1974): 106.

6. (p. 81) T. G. Parks, *Proceedings of the Royal Society of Medicine*, vol. 66, July 1973.
7. (p. 82) See note 1 above.

Notes, Chapter 9

1. (p. 88) Philip Rubin, "Current Concepts in Cancer, Introduction," *Journal of the American Medical Association* 231 (February 3, 1975): 513–516.
2. (p. 90) "Roughage In The Diet," *Medical World News* 15 (September 6, 1974): 35–42.
3. (p. 92) Benjamin H. Ershoff, "Antitoxic Effects of Plant Fiber," *American Journal of Clinical Nutrition* 27 (December 1974): 1395–1398.
4. (p. 94) See note 3 above.
5. (p. 95) William Haenszel, J.W. Berg et al, "Large-Bowel Cancer In Hawaiian Japanese," *Journal of the National Cancer Institute* 51 (December 1973): 1765–1779.
6. (p. 96) See note 5 above.
7. (p. 96) See note 5 above.
8. (p. 96) See note 5 above.
9. (p. 97) *New York Times*, 9 February 1974.
10. (p. 97) M.J. Hill et al, "Faecal Bile-Acids and Clostridia in Patients with Cancer of the Large Bowel," *Lancet* 1 (March 8, 1975): 535–539.
11. (p. 97) Hill, "Steroid Nuclear Dehydrogenation and Colon Cancer," *American Journal of Clinical Nutrition* 27 (December 1974): 1475–1480.
12. (p. 98) See note 11 above.
13. (p. 100) "Selenium May Give Protection Against Certain Carcinomas," *Medical Tribune*, 27 June 1973, p. 27.

Notes, Appendix C

1. (p. 134) Study conducted by Dr. Ira Shannon, Houston Veterans Administration Hospital, *Journal of Dentistry for Children*, September-October 1974.

Index

A

abdomen, pain in, diet and, 78
abdominal muscles, hemorrhoids and, 45, 46
abdominal pain, diet and, 78
acids, bile, beef and, 97–100
  cholesterol and, 51, 52
  fiber and, 52
Africans, bowel disease and, 3
  diet of, 3
apple crisp, 113
atherosclerosis, heart disease and, 50

B

baked tomatoes, 124
banana-nut bread, 111
bananas, diarrhea and, 40
  snackin', 113
beef, as carcinogen, 94–100
  bile acids and, 97–100
  bowel cancer and, 97–100. See also *cancer*.
bile acids, beef and, 97–100
  cholesterol and, 51, 52
  fiber and, 52
bowel cancer, beef and, 87. See also *cancer*.
bowel disease, Africans and, 3
  control of, 2, 3
incidence of, 2
bowel function, normalizers for, 38, 39
bowel movements, water and, 24, 25
bowels, function of, normalizers for, 38, 39
bran, advantages of, 13, 14
  as cereal, 13, 14
  as normalizer, 38
  calorie absorption and, 62, 63
  constipation and, 9, 10
  definition of, viii
  diarrhea and, 38–40
  diet of, benefits of, 78–82
  diverticulitis and, 82–85
  effects of, 13–15
  fiber and, 10, 13
  hot raisin, 117
  recipes for, 103–126
  sources of, 14, 35, 36
  taste of, 13
bran bread, 104
bran cake, carrot carob, 110
bran coffee, 107
bran cookies, 109
bran diet, benefits of, 78–82
bran English muffins, 106
bran muffins, 105
bran sesame crackers, 108
bread, banana-nut, 111